Degenerative Diseases of the Cervical Spine

Alexander König • Uwe Spetzger

Degenerative Diseases of the Cervical Spine

Therapeutic Management in the Subaxial Section

Springer

Alexander König
Department of Neurosurgery
Klinikum Karlsruhe
Karlsruhe, Baden-Württemberg
Germany

Uwe Spetzger
Department of Neurosurgery
Klinikum Karlsruhe
Karlsruhe, Baden-Württemberg
Germany

ISBN 978-3-319-47297-3 ISBN 978-3-319-47298-0 (eBook)
DOI 10.1007/978-3-319-47298-0

Library of Congress Control Number: 2016962085

Printed on acid-free paper

This Springer imprint is published by Springer Nature
The registered company is Springer International Publishing AG
The registered company address is Gewerbestrasse 11, 6330 Cham, Switzerland

Foreword

The high practical relevance as well as the comprehensible and rich illustrated presentation in our book is supposed to be a guide for the conservative and particularly surgical treatment of degenerative diseases of the cervical spine in the daily clinical practice.

The chapters about basics and indications for surgery are addressed to beginners. For advanced spine surgeons, probably the chapters about approaches, choice of implants and surgical techniques are of primary interest.

Especially the growing number and variety of implants for the replacement of intervertebral discs and vertebral bodies are a big challenge for the spine surgeon since medical benefit and economical aspects have to be considered. In this book, we would like to give some help in the decision-making process about the surgical indication and the choice of a certain implant based on scientific findings and personal experience. It has been our aim to demonstrate this practically with many figures as well as systematically and clearly at the same time.

We would like to thank Mrs. Joanna Renwick and Mr. Andre Tournois from Springer for the continuous and prompt support at every stage of the book project.

In particular, we thank our families for the ongoing understanding and support during the time-consuming work on this project.

Karlsruhe, July 2016 Alexander König and Uwe Spetzger

Preface

The book by König and Spetzger is a modern and practical compendium for the experienced as well as for the beginner in the field of surgical treatment of degenerative diseases of the cervical spine. The chapters about anatomical and physiological basics as well as those about indications for surgery are primarily addressed to trainees. The chapters about surgical approaches, biomechanical considerations during the choice of implants and surgical techniques are of interest for advanced spine surgeons.

Like in a good 'cookbook', each single step of surgery is illustrated by perfect intraoperative photographic images. Several microsurgical techniques are shown, and important practical hints are given for the different types of implants. The consecutive and clear figurative demonstration of the particular operations provides a well-defined surgical strategy to the reader. Herefrom results a didactically valuable and very practical surgical textbook.

Nowadays, the market of implants for cervical spine surgery is almost unmanageable and still growing. Due to their surgical experience which is referred to the reader, the authors give support for the choice of implants based on biomechanical, strategical and safety-related aspects.

The book is a must-have for every spine surgeon treating patients with degenerative diseases of the cervical spine.

Phoenix, Arizona, USA Volker K. H. Sonntag, MD, Professor of Clinical Surgery

Contents

1 Introduction

The current trend in cervical spinal surgery is affected by continuous optimisation of intervertebral cages and disc prostheses. The latter have been developed since the 1990s based on experiences with lumbar prostheses. The initial focus was put on different designs with titanium endplates and a plastic core. Nowadays, there is a development of single unit implants made of elastic polymeric material. To what extent these implants provide an approximation to physiological conditions in shape, function and bony anchorage is still unclear.

1.1 Background

During the last decade, the number of surgeries for the treatment of degenerative diseases of the cervical spine has continuously increased. This development is based on an increasing life expectance as well as on the improvement of diagnostic and therapeutical options.

Furthermore, the number of available implants for the replacement of a removed intervertebral disc has exponentially increased. This development can be seen for dynamic implants (disc prostheses) as well as for non-dynamic implants (so-called cages). Because of the relatively short period since their introduction to the market, numerous implants have been evaluated on the basis of small patient populations and short follow-up times only. Furthermore, there are a relatively small number of studies with radiological and clinical comparison of fusion versus total disc replacement. In terms of choosing a certain implant, there are different algorithms depending on the surgeon's preferences. Nevertheless, most surgeons include patient's age, range of motion of the affected level, range of motion of adjacent levels and the number of affected levels in their decision-making process.

There is a similar situation for cervical vertebral body replacement in cases of confluent multilevel stenoses. The interposition of an iliac crest bone graft is still the

A. König, U. Spetzger, *Degenerative Diseases of the Cervical Spine*,
DOI 10.1007/978-3-319-47298-0_1

gold standard, but there are also implants made of polyetheretherketone as well as of titanium on the market. The use of a certain material differs between institutions analogue to disc replacement.

Furthermore, different spine surgeons prefer different approaches and instrumentations at the cervical spine (anterior, posterior, combined) in cases of spinal instability.

The aim of this book is to explain the strategies in choosing a surgical approach and an implant for disc or vertebral body replacement based on the authors´ experiences and recent biomechanical and clinical studies.

1.2 History of Diagnostics and Therapy of Cervical Disc Herniation

The etiological relation between disc degeneration and spondylosis deformans was first described by Wenzel (1824). A cervical spondylosis as the reason for radicular symptoms was identified by Braun (1875). In the early twentieth century, a cervical disc herniation as a possible reason of paraparesis (thus myelopathic symptoms) was recognised (Hawk 1936). Küttner probably was the first surgeon removing a cervical disc herniation that compressed a nerve root (Frykholm 1969). In the 1930s and 1940s, numerous publications reported about the clinical significance of discogenic nerve root and spinal cord compression. At that time cervical disc herniations were removed using a laminectomy or hemilaminectomy. Since these methods did not result in radicular decompression in the intervertebral foramen, Scoville (1946) as well as Frykholm (1947) developed surgical techniques for foraminal nerve root decompression using a drill. Despite the modification of the posterior surgical techniques, it was not possible to achieve sufficient treatment of medial osteophytes or disc herniations. Therefore, Cloward (1958) developed an alternative method using an anterior approach. After anterior discectomy, a spondylodesis with a cylindric iliac crest bone graft was performed. Robinson and Smith (1958) introduced a similar technique that used a rectangular autologous bone graft. In the 1980s, the anterior plating was established to avoid local complications with the bone graft (Caspar et al. 1989).

Because of the morbidity at the site of harvesting the iliac bone graft, Grote and Rottgen (1967) introduced polymethylmethacrylate (PMMA) as an alternative to the autologous transplant. PMMA is still used at some institutions, but critics of this technique point to the increased rate of pseudarthrosis and heat during the polymerisation process. For this reason, the industry developed intervertebral cages that have become the standard implant worldwide. Usually these cages have a central hole that enables bony fusion especially when filled with osteoinductive material. The idea of using intervertebral cages came from veterinary medicine (DeBowes et al. 1984; Bagby 1988) because cervical fusion is indicated in horses suffering from the Wobbler syndrome which is a veterinary disease with gait ataxia due to spondylotic myelopathy.

Since the 1990s, the use of intervertebral cages for cervical fusion increased continuously. They are made of either titanium, carbon or polyetheretherketone (PEEK). Titanium cages are produced in a way that enlarges the surface of the cage leading to a better osseointegration. Compared to PEEK cages, they are supposed to lead to worse results in terms of clinical results as well as maintaining the intervertebral height and angle of lordosis (Chen et al. 2013). The main disadvantage of titanium cages is the massive artefacts they produce during MR imaging. Thus, the nonrestrictive assessment of MR images is the essential advantage of PEEK cages.

Due to the further development of surgical treatment of cervical disc herniation with a microsurgical nerve root or spinal cord decompression, usually an effective pain relief and neurological recovery is achieved. After the continuous improvement of surgical results, the maintenance of motion at the affected level came into the focus of research and development. The main argument for maintaining motion at a decompressed level is to avoid accelerated degeneration at adjacent levels. This is supposed to be achieved by pursuing physiological patterns of motion (Le et al. 2004).

In the early 1980s, the development of lumbar disc prostheses began. The most frequently used implant was the lumbar SB Charité prosthesis (Büttner-Janz et al. 1989) that was the first total disc replacement achieving an FDA (Food and Drug Administration) approval.

Besides the continuous further development of implants, the invasiveness and morbidity of cervical disc surgery were reduced by the introduction of the operating microscope in the 1980s.

With increasing therapeutical success of lumbar total disc replacement, the development of cervical prostheses began in the 1990s. Early implants like the Cummins-Bristol artificial cervical joint or the Frenchay cervical disc (later called Prestige) had a metal-on-metal design and were fixed with screws in the vertebral bodies. A maintenance of motion was achieved but there were screw disc locations and breakings observed (Le et al. 2004). In the late 1990s, the Bryan disc was introduced being the first device with a metal-on-plastic design based on two titanium endplates with a polyurethane core. For the Bryan disc, prospective studies reported about good clinical results and adequate maintenance of motion (Bryan 2002). Nevertheless, for the implantation of the Bryan disc, the use of complex surgical instruments was necessary, and the dissection of the intervertebral space with a drill leads to an increased rate of heterotopic ossification.

After the success of the lumbar device ProDisc-L, the development of the cervical ProDisc-C began. This prosthesis was made of two metal-polyethylene components that made up a ball-in-socket design. Critics of this kind of design argue that it does not mimic the physiological motion of the cervical spine with its variable centre of rotation that changes its position especially during flexion/extension and lateral bending by doing a translational motion. This pattern of motion is supposed to be achieved by novel designs with loose components that move against each other (Mobi-C prosthesis) or plastic analogues of annulus and nucleus (M6C prosthesis). Furthermore, there was a potential higher complication rate for the ProDisc-C because it was necessary to create gutters in the endplates with a special chisel.

The latest generation of cervical total disc replacement is made up by single-unit implants like the freedom cervical disc or the Cadisc-C although the latter is not produced anymore. Furthermore, there is a lack of prospective multicentre studies with a high number of patients to evaluate these implants. An important aspect in the long-term results for these expensive implants will be the rate of heterotopic ossification and consecutive bony fusion which leads to a loss of their function. With more long-term results for the different implant designs, the high number of available implants on the market will probably be reduced.

References

Bagby GW. Arthrodesis by the distraction-compression method using a stainless steel implant. Orthopedics. 1988;11(6):931–4.

Braun J. Klinische und anatomische Beiträge zur Kenntnis der Spondylitis deformans als einer der häufigsten Ursachen mannigfacher Neurosen, namentlich der Spinalirritation. Hannover: Carl Rümpler; 1875.

Bryan Jr VE. Cervical motion segment replacement. Eur Spine J. 2002;11 Suppl 2:S92–7.

Büttner-Janz K, Schellnack K, Zippel H. Biomechanics of the SB Charité lum- bar intervertebral disc endoprosthesis. Int Orthop. 1989;13(3):173–6.

Caspar W, Barbier DD, Klara PM. Anterior cervical fusion and Caspar plate stabilisation for cervical trauma. Neurosurgery. 1989;25:491–502.

Chen Y, Wang X, Lu X, et al. Comparison of titanium and polyetheretherke- tone (PEEK) cages in the surgical treatment of multilevel cervical spondylotic myelopathy: a prospective, randomized, control study with over 7-year follow-up. Eur Spine J. 2013;22(7):1539–46.

Cloward RB. The anterior approach for removal of ruptured cervical disks. J Neurosurg. 1958;15(6):602–17.

DeBowes RM, Grant BD, Bagby GW, et al. Cervical vertebral interbody fusion in the horse: a comparative study of bovine xenografts and autografts sup- ported by stainless steel baskets. Am J Vet Res. 1984;45(1):191–9.

Frykholm R. Deformities of dural pouches and strictures of dural sheaths in the cervical regionproducing nerve-root compression. A contribution to the etiology and operative treatment of brachial neuralgia. J Neurosurg. 1947;4:403–13.

Frykholm R. Die cervicalen Bandscheibenschäden. In: Olivecrona H, Tönnis W, editors. Handbuch der Neurochirurgie. Siebenter Band/Erster Teil. Berlin/New York: Springer; 1969.

Grote W, Röttgen P. Die ventrale Fusion bei der zervikalen Osteochondrose und ihre Behandlungsergebnisse. Acta Neurochir. 1967;16:218–40.

Hawk WA. Spinal compression caused by ecchochondrosis of the intraverte- bral fibrocartilage: with a review of the recent literature. Brain. 1936;59:202–24.

Le H, Thongtrangan I, Kim DH. Historical review of cervical arthroplasty. Neurosurg Focus. 2004;17(3):E1.

Robinson RA, Smith GW. The treatment of certain cervical spine disorders by anterior removal of the intervertebral disc and interbody fusion. J Bone Joint Surg Am. 1958;40-A(3):607–24.

Scoville WB. Contribution to discussion about ruptured cervical discs. Arch Neurol Psychiatr. 1946;56:722–3.

Wenzel C. Über die Krankheiten am Rückgrathe. Bamberg: W. L. Wesche; 1824.

Anatomical Aspects

2

The cervical spine has an exceptional position within spine surgery because of its filigree dimensions and its relations to numerous neurovascular structures. Knowledge of dimensions of vertebrae and discs is an essential precondition for surgical procedures with implantation of cages, prostheses or vertebral body replacements. Topographical anatomical relations are of great importance for the several surgical approaches.

2.1 Dimensions

The cervical spine is the most moveable and filigree part of the human spine. It is surrounded by numerous neurovascular structures: vertebral arteries, carotid arteries, nerve roots of the spinal cord and prevertebral ganglions. An overview over the dimensions of the seven cervical vertebrae as well as the medium heights of the cervical discs is given in Fig. 2.1 (Lang 1991).

2.2 Vertebral Body, Intervertebral Disc and Uncinate Process

The cervical vertebrae 3–7 have a shape that is typical for the cervical spine (Fig. 2.2). The cervical vertebrae 1 and 2 (atlas and axis) have morphological and functional exceptional position because of their importance for movements of the head. The condyles of the squama occipitalis together with the cranial articular surfaces of the atlas form the atlanto-occipital joint (C0/C1) which is a big range of motion for flexion/extension. Atlas and axis form the atlantoaxial joint (C1/C2) which has a high degree of rotational ability. The functional level between axis and third cervical vertebra (C2/C3) enables a large amount of lateral flexion. The subaxial cervical

A. König, U. Spetzger, *Degenerative Diseases of the Cervical Spine*,
DOI 10.1007/978-3-319-47298-0_2

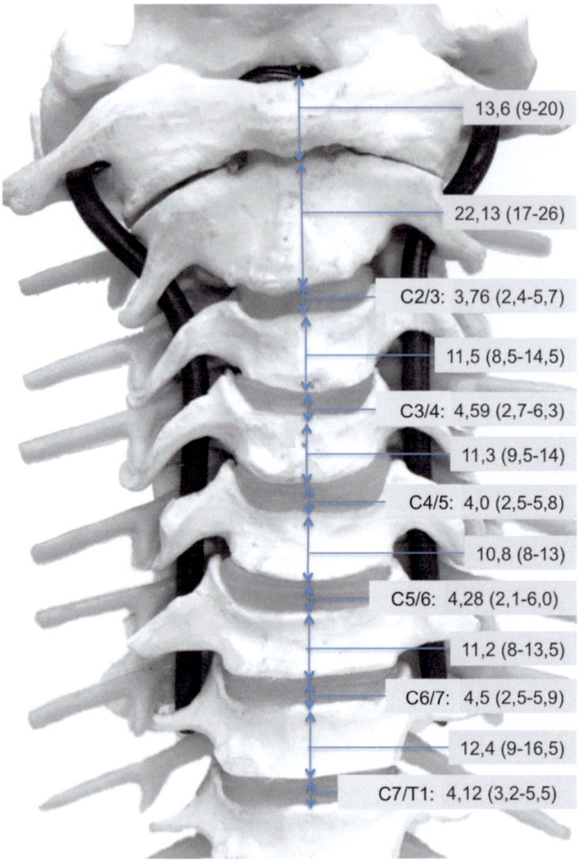

Fig. 2.1 Average height of cervical vertebrae and intervertebral discs

spine from the third to the seventh vertebra shows a wide morphological homogeneity which reflects in the similar range of motion of the levels C3/C4 to C6/C7 (Table 3.1).

A morphological special characteristic of the cervical spine is the uncinate process (Fig. 2.3) which is located at the cranial lateral aspects of the vertebral bodies. It limits rotational movements and provides integrity of the neuroforamen during lateral bending (Tubbs 2012). The upper uncinate processes a lateral orientation only, and the lower ones a dorsal orientation (Lang 1991).

The intervertebral discs being deformable units fill the intervertebral spaces. Movements of vertebrae against each other base on an interaction of intervertebral discs and intervertebral joints (articulationes intervertebrales; see Sect. 2.3).

The intervertebral discs ensure the elasticity of the spinal column and work as a shock absorber (Lang 1991). The outer fibrous ring (anulus

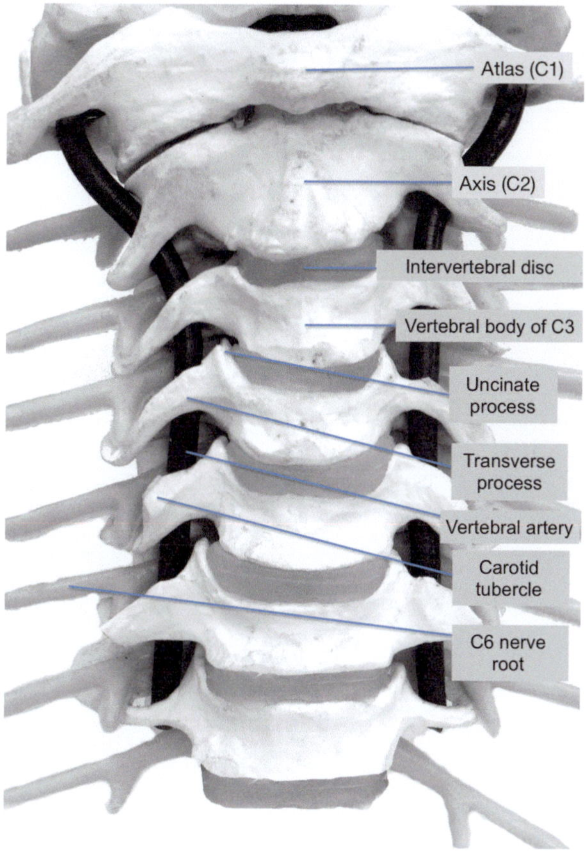

Fig. 2.2 Anatomy of the cervical spine. Ventral view with the most relevant anatomical structures

fibrosus) of the intervertebral disc surrounds the inner gel-like centre (nucleus pulposus) and consists of collagenous (90 %) and elastic (10 %) fibres (Fig. 2.2; Lang (1991).

2.3 Vertebral Arch and Facet Joints

The vertebral arches together with the segmental ligamenta flava form the dorsal limitation of the spinal canal and thus protect the spinal cord. The intervertebral joints (zygapophyseal joints) are often called facet joints in the clinical practice and are synovial joint between the superior articular process of one vertebra and the inferior articular process of the adjacent cranial vertebra (Fig. 2.3). The function of each pair of facet joints is the guidance and limitation of segmental motion (Frykholm 1969; Milne 1993).

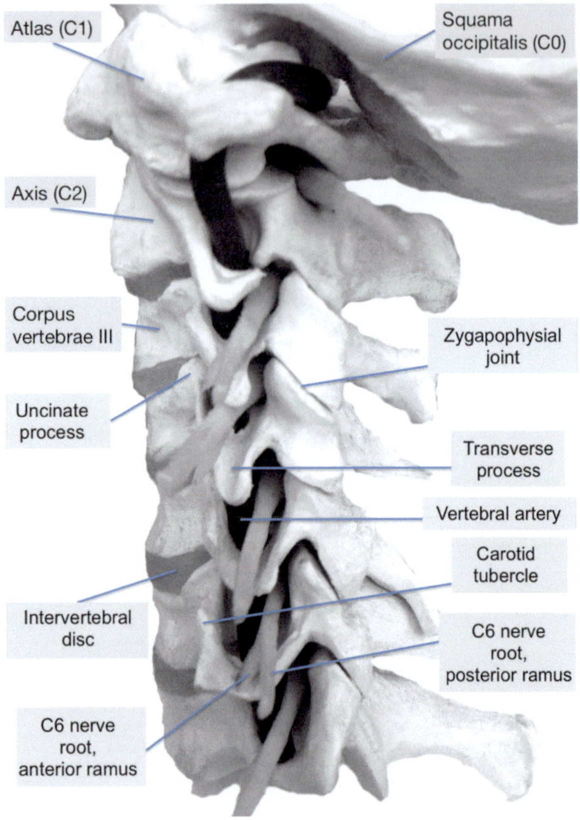

Fig. 2.3 Anatomy of the cervical spine. Lateral view with the most relevant anatomical structures

2.4 Cervical Muscles

2.4.1 Ventral Muscles

The superficial layer of ventral cervical muscles consists of the platysma which is innervated by the facial nerve and belongs to the mimic muscles. The bilateral sternocleidomastoid muscles are underneath and turn the head when only one of them is activated. When activated on both sides, they lift the head and pull it a bit anteriorly with extension of the upper cervical spine at the same time (Fig. 2.4).

When using the anterolateral standard approach to the cervical spine, the omohyoid muscle is pushed medially. This muscle tenses the cervical fascia. The anterior scalene, middle scalene and posterior scalene muscles are located at the lateral aspect of the cervical spine. They bend it laterally and lift the first rib during inspiration.

The deepest layer of muscles at the ventral aspect of the cervical spine consists of the rectus capitis anterior muscle, longus capitis muscle and longus colli muscle. All of the three muscles provide anterior flexion and ipsilateral rotation.

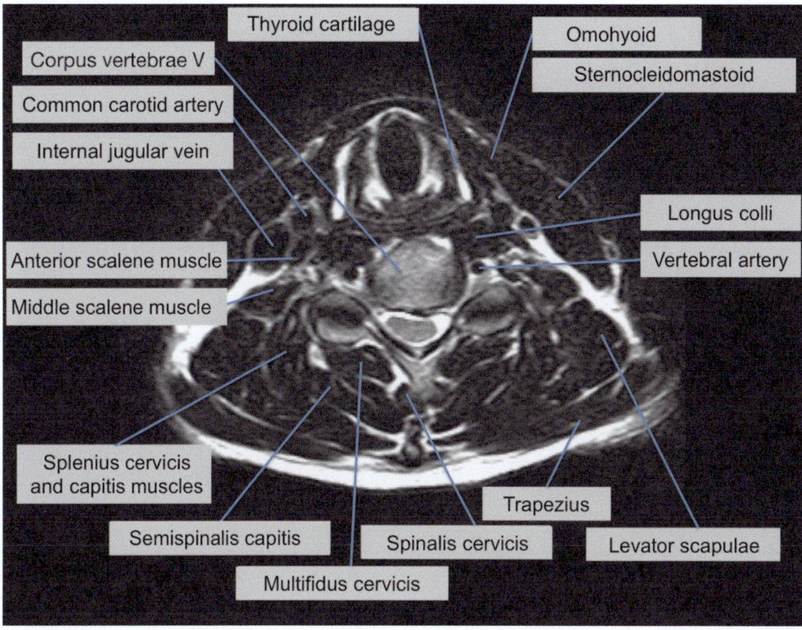

Fig. 2.4 Axial cross section (T2-weighted MR image) at the level of the inferior part of the fifth cervical vertebra showing the most important muscles for spinal motion

2.4.2 Dorsal Muscles

The muscles of the neck are covered by the trapezius muscle. It has numerous effects on shoulder girdle and arms. At the spinal column, it causes flattening of the thoracic kyphosis. Underneath we find the splenius cervicis and splenius capitis muscles. During unilateral activation they provide lateral bending and ipsilateral rotation. Activation on both sides leads to dorsal extension of the cervical spine. The deeper located muscles (semispinalis capitis and semispinalis cervicis muscles, longissimus capitis and longissimus cervicis muscles) have an identical function.

At the tips of the spinous processes, the spinalis capitis and cervicis muscles can be found which provide lateral bending when activated unilaterally and dorsal extension when activated bilaterally.

Analogue to the thoracic and lumbar spine, the cervical spine is guided by multifidi muscles that rotate the head to the opposite side when activated unilaterally. Activation on both sides leads to dorsal extension (Fig. 2.4).

Fine-tuning of head motion is provided by small and deep muscles between the levels C0/C1 and C2/C3: major and minor rectus capitis muscles (extension), superior and inferior obliquus capitis muscles (lateral bending and extension) and lateral rectus capitis muscles (lateral bending).

Except the trapezius muscle, all of the muscles mentioned above belong to the autochthonous musculature of the neck.

2.5 Topographic Anatomy

2.5.1 Anterior Approach

In the majority of cases with cervical disc herniation or narrowing of the spinal canal, the anterolateral standard approach is the adequate surgical approach to the cervical spine (see Sect. 7.1). The most important anatomical structures in the surgical field during the several steps of surgery are shown in Figs. 2.5, 2.6, 2.7, 2.8 and 2.9.

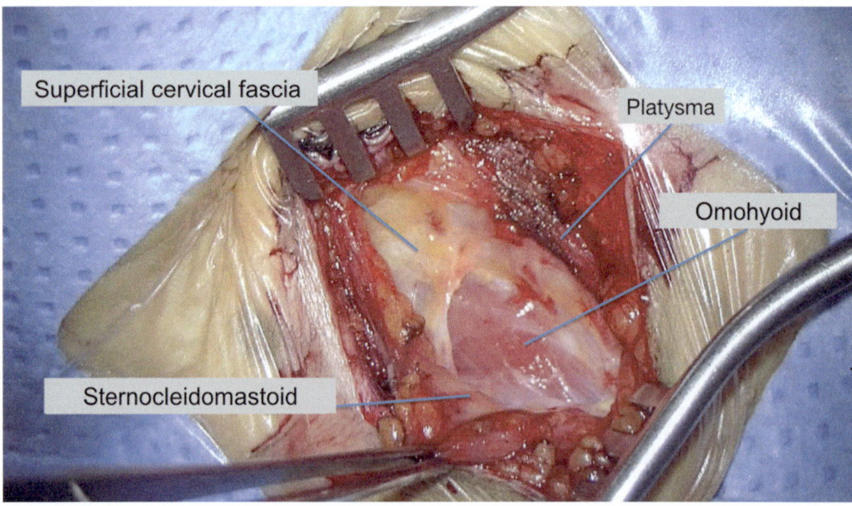

Fig. 2.5 Anatomy in the surgical field after skin incision and transection of the platysma

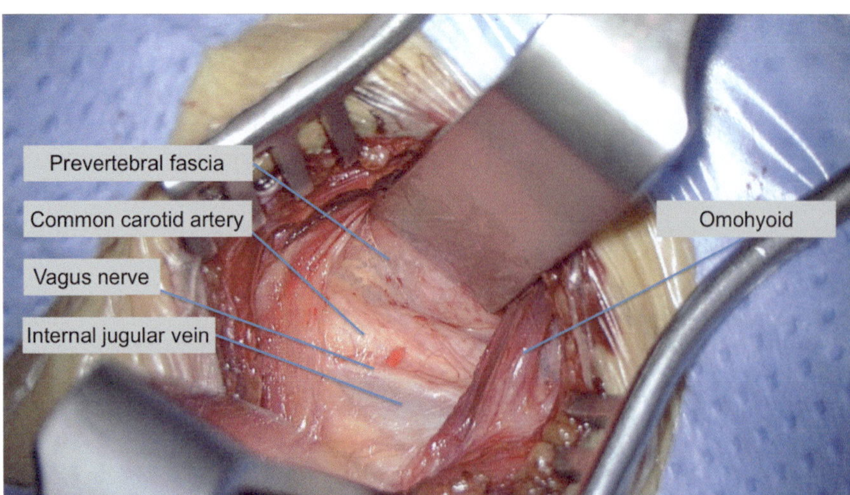

Fig. 2.6 Location of the internal jugular vein, carotid artery and vagus nerve after medial retraction of the straight cervical muscles

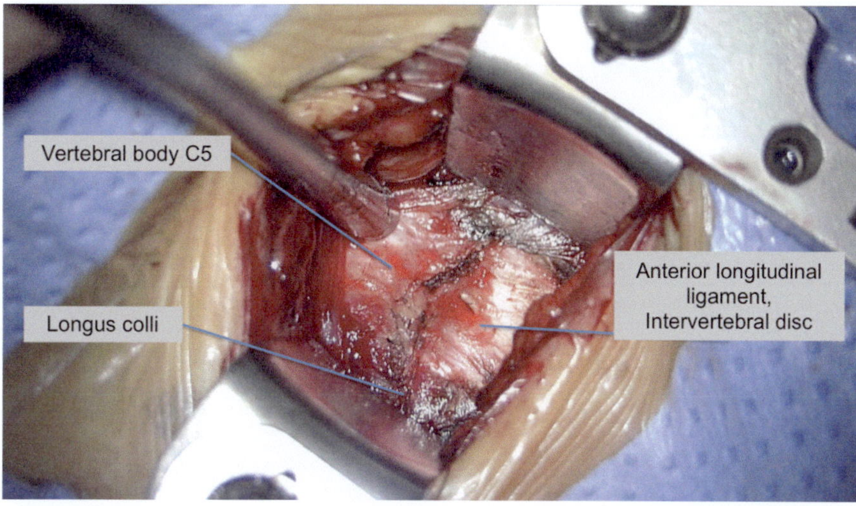

Fig. 2.7 Ventral surface of the cervical spine after lateral retraction of the internal jugular vein, carotid artery and vagus nerve as well as medial retraction of the oesophagus and trachea

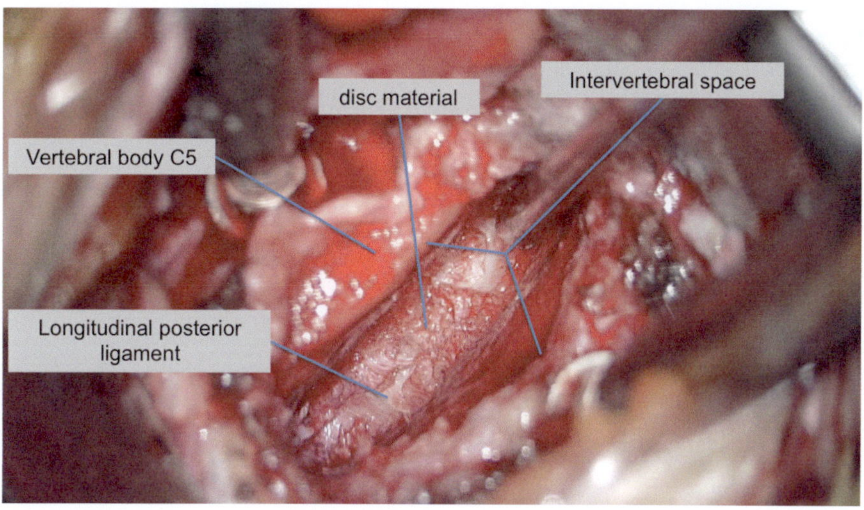

Fig. 2.8 Surgical field and anatomical structures after subtotal discectomy

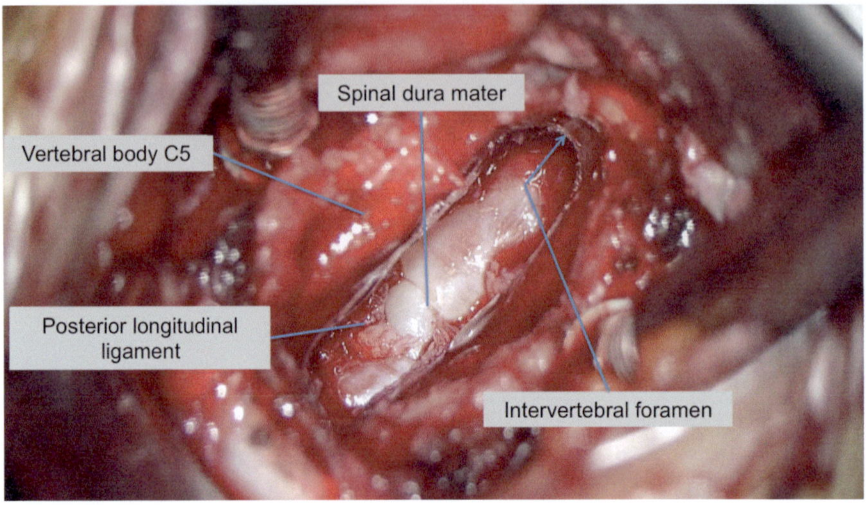

Fig. 2.9 Situation after discectomy and partial resection of the posterior longitudinal ligament

2.5.2 Posterior Approach

A laminectomy and/or dorsal spondylodesis is done by using a nuchal midline approach. The most important anatomical structures in the surgical field during the several steps of surgery are shown in Figs. 2.10, 2.11, 2.12, 2.13 and 2.14.

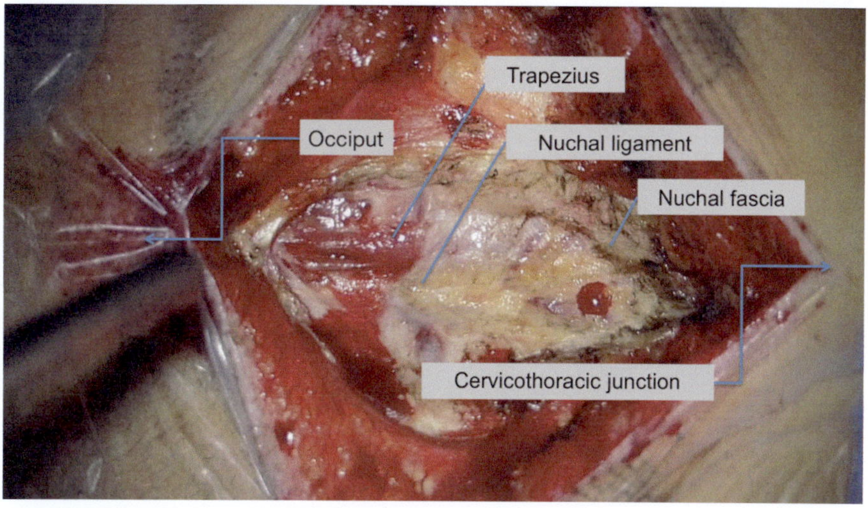

Fig. 2.10 Surgical field after craniocaudal skin incision and transection of the fascia in the midline

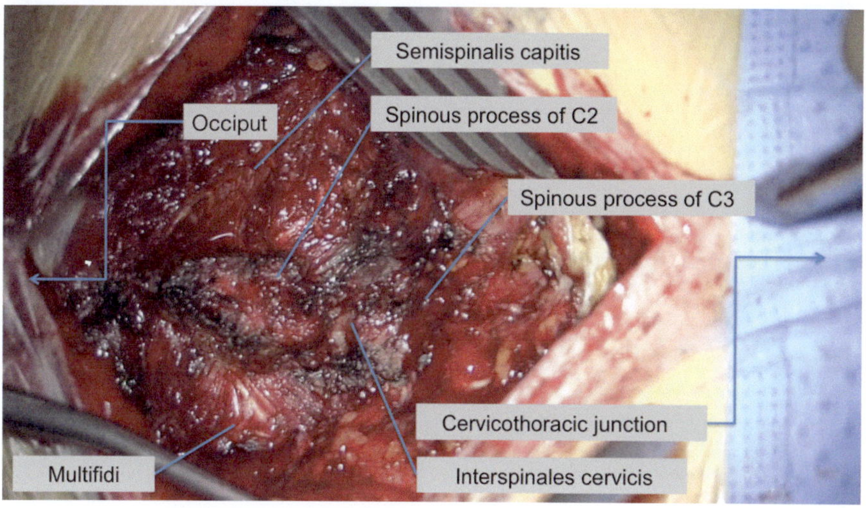

Fig. 2.11 Surgical field after transection of the ligamentum nuchae in the midline and exposure of the spinous processes of the second and third cervical vertebra

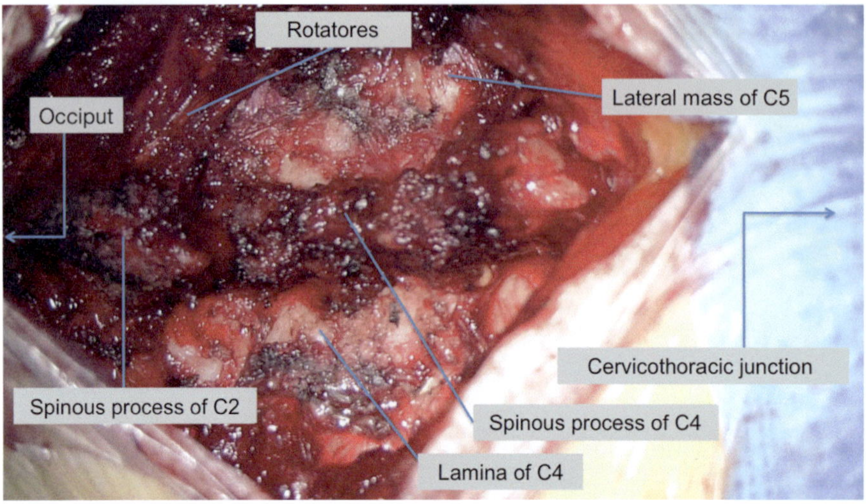

Fig. 2.12 Surgical field after dissection of all muscles from the laminae of C3 to C6

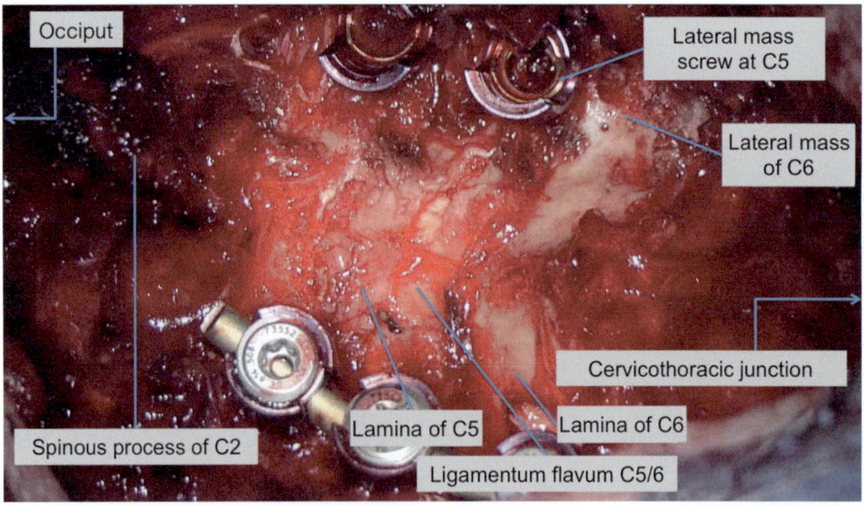

Fig. 2.13 Surgical field after removal of the spinous processes of C4 to C6 and partially of C3. The ligamenta flava can be easily identified between the laminae

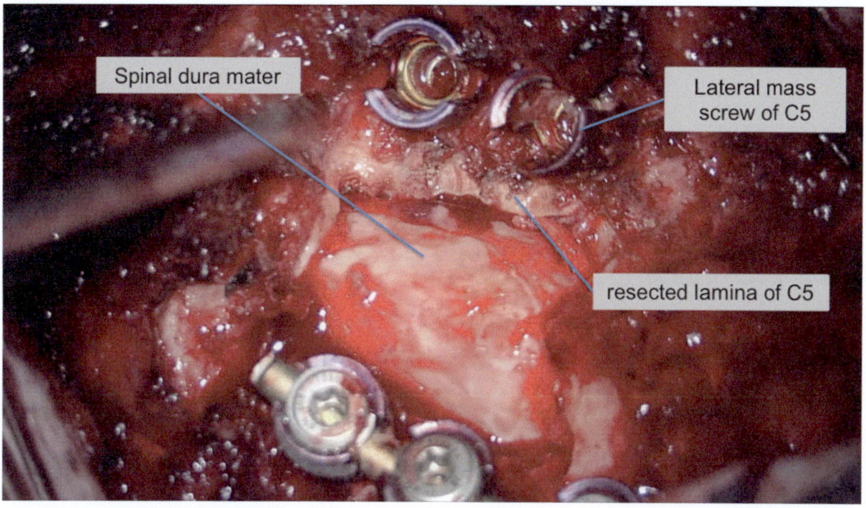

Fig. 2.14 Surgical field after decompression of the spinal canal by performing a laminectomy of C4 and C5

References

Frykholm R Die cervicalen Bandscheibenschäden. In: Olivecrona H, Tönnis W (Hrsg.) Handbuch der Neurochirurgie. Siebenter Band/Erster Teil. Springer, Berlin/Heidelberg/New York; 1969

Lang J. Klinische Anatomie der Halswirbelsäule. Stuttgart/New York: Thieme; 1991.

Milne N. Composite motion in cervical disc segments. Clin Biochem. 1993;8(4):193–202.

Tubbs RS, Rompala OJ, Verma K, Mortazavi MM, Benninger B, Loukas M, Chambers MR. Analysis of the uncinate processes of the cervical spine: an anatomical study. J Neurosurg Spine. 2012;16(4):402–7.

Biomechanical Aspects

3

The cervical spine is the most flexible part of the spinal column with six degrees of freedom in total. Every motion segment makes up a complex balanced system which enables several functions: posture with simultaneous flexibility, balance by providing compensation movements, bearing of axial loads and protection of the spinal cord. The biomechanical spinal research uses more and more the principle of finite elements. Furthermore, the latest implants for total disc replacement have to be tested in terms of their in vivo kinematics.

3.1 Motions of the Cervical Spine

The cervical spine enables motion in six different directions:

- Anterior flexion and posterior extension (inclination and reclination of the head) in the sagittal plane
- Lateral bending to the left and right in the coronal plane
- Rotation to the left and right in the axial plane

Motions of the cervical spine under physiological conditions are usually combinations of these basic movements. A special feature is the fact that additionally to the actual motion (e.g. flexion/extension in the sagittal plane), the instantaneous centre of rotation (ICR) dynamically changes within the disc. Thus, there is an additional translation movement. This phenomenon hast to be considered in the design of artificial discs for total disc replacement. Furthermore, Lee (1997) could show that there is a displacement of the ICR in cases of spinal instability.

A synopsis of the range of motion of the cervical levels in the different planes is given in Table 3.1.

The physiological shape of the cervical spine in the neutral position is a lordosis which means an arrangement of the vertebrae with a dorsal concavity in the sagittal plane.

A. König, U. Spetzger, *Degenerative Diseases of the Cervical Spine*,
DOI 10.1007/978-3-319-47298-0_3

Table 3.1 Segmental motion of the cervical spine with mean values and minimum/maximum (angle degrees); Panjabi and White (1990)

Direction of motion	C2/3	C3/4	C4/5	C5/6	C6/7	Whole cervical spine
Flexion/extension	10 (5–16)	15 (7–26)	20 (13–29)	20 13–29)	17 (6–26)	75
Unilateral bending	10 (7–20)	11 (9–15)	11 (0–16)	8 (0–16)	7 (0–17)	35
Unilateral axial rotation	3 (0–10)	7 (3–10)	7 (1–12)	7 (2–12)	6 (2–10)	45

3.2 The Functional Spinal Unit and Its Function

One cervical spinal motion segment is considered as the smallest functional spinal unit (FSU). The FSU consists of two adjacent vertebrae including facet joints, intervertebral disc, anterior and posterior longitudinal ligament, interspinous ligament as well as the autochthonous muscles. These anatomical components make up a complex balanced system that enables the basic functions of the spine:

- Upright posture with simultaneous flexibility
- Balance by providing compensational movements
- Bearing of axial loads and compression stresses
- Protection of the spinal cord

The first two functions are provided by the neuromuscular system of the spinal column (autochthonous muscles and their innervation). After the perception of movements or a change of position, the autochthonous muscles receive triggers from spinocerebellar tracts that finally lead to a continuous muscular stabilisation of the spinal column. The necessary flexibility of the functional spinal unit is provided by the elastic intervertebral disc in the anterior section and the facet joints in the posterior section.

3.3 Bearing of Loads by the Spinal Column

3.3.1 Intervertebral Disc

Axial loads are mainly absorbed by the intervertebral discs. Compression leads to distortion of the nucleus pulposus that tensions the anulus fibrosus. The latter consists of tight and elastic fibres that finally absorb axial load on the intervertebral disc. By doing this, they ensure that the intervertebral disc finally reaches its original shape (White and Panjabi 1990). During physiological motions of the spine (flexion, extension, lateral bending, axial rotation), the intervertebral disc is affected by compressive, distractive, rotational and shearing forces. As mentioned above, the axial loads are mainly absorbed by the nucleus pulposus. Rotational and shearing forces are mainly compensated by the anulus fibrosus and its kind and configuration of fibres.

3.3.2 Vertebrae

The biomechanical function of the vertebra with its trabecular bone structure is taking compressive axial forces. Because of the anatomical structure of a vertebra, the vertebral body takes 80 % and the facet joints 20 % of axial loads (Kirkaldy-Willis 1990). A loss of bone density in the second half of life leads to a decrease of compression stability of the vertebral body. A reduction of bone mass of already 25 % causes a decrease of compression stability of 50 % (Kirkaldy-Willis 1990).

The orientation of facet joints at the middle and lower cervical spine is 45° to the sagittal plane (Lang 1991); thus, lateral bending to one side leads to rotation of spinous processes to the opposite side. Flexion and extension are linked to horizontal translation (White 1990).

Flexion and extension are mainly done between the fourth and sixth cervical vertebra. Lateral bending is mainly provided by the functional spinal units between the third and fifth vertebra. The main part of rotation (more than 50 % of the whole cervical spine) is provided by atlas and axis due to their special shape (White and Panjabi 1990).

3.3.3 Ligaments

The spinal ligamentous system withstands tension forces and transfers movements between vertebrae with the tension resistance of the anterior longitudinal ligament being twice as high as of the posterior longitudinal ligament. A specialty of the ligamentum flavum which is a segmental ligament is its main consistence of elastin (80 %). It has a high tension in rest when the spinal column is in a neutral position. This tension increases the tension of the intervertebral disc in rest which finally leads to a higher stability of the functional spinal unit (Raabe 1997).

3.3.4 Instability

For the concept of segmental instability, the anatomical structures of the cervical spine are divided into anterior and posterior elements. Anterior elements are vertebral bodies, intervertebral discs, transverse processes as well as anterior and posterior longitudinal ligaments. Posterior elements are vertebral arches, facet joints, spinous processes, interspinous processes and ligamenta flava.

Biomechanical instability is defined as an increased, abnormal mobility with pathological movement patterns. Clinical instability is characterised by local pain and/or signs of nerve root or spinal cord compression (Raabe 1997).

White and Panjabi (1990) defined main criteria for spinal instability:

- Injury of anterior elements
- Injury of posterior elements
- Positive stretch test
- Translation in the sagittal plane more than 3.5 mm or 20 %
- Rotation in the sagittal plane more than 20 degrees
- Relative angulation in the sagittal plane of more than 11 degrees
- Spinal cord injury

Furthermore, these authors mentioned several side criteria:

- Congenital narrow spinal canal (less than 13 mm)
- Abnormal low height of the intervertebral disc
- Nerve root injury

White and Panjabi made up a checklist by the means of those criteria for the diagnosis of instability in the middle and lower cervical spine but it did not reach wide acceptance among clinical users. Nevertheless, most of the criteria mentioned above are nowadays used to assess instability of the cervical spine in MR images or functional X-ray images.

3.3.5 Biomechanical Analytical Methods

During the last decades, research concerning the biomechanical properties of the cervical spine was mainly based on the use of cadaveric specimen. This kind of research brought useful information about the behaviour of the intervertebral discs, but nevertheless the informative value of cadaveric studies is limited concerning the biomechanical properties of the whole cervical spine because there is a lack of functioning muscles that stabilise the spinal column. Therefore, finite element model studies have become more and more important during the last decade because the biomechanical properties of vertebrae, intervertebral discs and muscles can be reproduced with the help of computer software. Furthermore, different implants can be reproduced including their effect on adjacent levels (Hussain 2013).

Another challenge for biomechanical research concerning the cervical spine is the fact that the results of in vitro and in vivo studies after total disc replacement significantly differ from each other. Therefore, Goel et al. (2011) requested a forced research in the field of in vivo kinematics after total disc replacement.

References

Goel VK, Faizan A, Palepu V, Bhattacharya S. Parameters that effect spine biomechanics following cervical disc replacement. Eur Spine J. 2011;21(Suppl 5):S688–99.

Hussain M, Nassr A, Natarajan RN, et al. Biomechanics of adjacent segments after a multilevel cervical corpectomy using anterior, posterior, and combined anterior-posterior instrumentation techniques: a finite element model study. Spine J. 2013;13(6):689–96.

Kirkaldy-Willis WH, Dupuis PR, Yong-Hing K. Biomechanics and ageing of the spine. In: Youmans JR, editor. Neurological Surgery. 3rd ed. Philadelphia: WB Saunders; 1990.
Lang J. Klinische Anatomie der Halswirbelsäule. Stuttgart New York: Thieme; 1991.
Lee SW, Draper ER, Hughes SP. Instantaneous center of rotation and instability of the cervical spine. A clinical study. Spine. 1997;22(6):641–7.
Raabe A, Wahler M. Biomechanics of the spine. In: Palmer JD, editor. Manual of neurosurgery. New York: Churchill Livingstone; 1997.
White III AA, Panjabi MM. Clinical biomechanics of the spine. Second ed. Philadelphia: J.B. Lippincott Comp; 1990.

4 Preoperative Diagnostics and Indication for Surgery

Past medical history and clinical examination give information about radicular and myelopathic symptoms and help to assess the acuity of clinical complaints and thus the urgency of a possible surgical treatment. MRI is the imaging method of first choice in cases of degenerative diseases of the cervical spine with neurological symptoms. The meaning of pre- and postoperative functional X-ray imaging has continuously increased because of the growing number of dynamic implants for total disc replacement. With the help of CT scans especially bony driven stenoses of the cervical spinal canal can be diagnosed in detail. A myelogram is useful in selected cases of multilevel narrowing of the spinal canal, especially in cases of previous surgeries. If it is impossible to confirm or exclude the indication for surgery by means of clinical complaints and imaging findings, it might be useful to consider electrophysiological techniques for the clinical diagnosis.

4.1 Past Medical History and Clinical Examination

4.1.1 General Considerations

The clinical symptoms of the patient are first and foremost when indicating surgery or not. There is a consensus that in cases of an acute palsy (hours or a few days) of muscles of the upper limb of grade 3 or less due to cervical disc herniation, surgical treatment is urgently indicated. In the rare case of acute tetraparesis (incomplete in most cases), there is even an emergency indication for surgical decompression of the spinal cord.

In the daily clinical routine, most patients suffer from recurrent neck pain and brachialgia or headaches as well as from sensory disorders of the upper limbs. Thus,

A. König, U. Spetzger, *Degenerative Diseases of the Cervical Spine*,
DOI 10.1007/978-3-319-47298-0_4

the main problem is the acute or chronic pain. In some of the patients, clinical examination shows a slight paresis of a certain muscle of the upper limb. If duration, intensity and resistance to therapy of clinical complaints heavily impair the patient's quality of life, elective surgical treatment can be recommended.

In cases of long-lasting compression of neural structures (months or years), the development of a somatoform disorder is possible due to the activation of the pain memory. That means that even after a decompression of nerves, thus after removing the morphological reason for the pain, a perception of pain persists. This fact should be considered in cases of complaints over months when the arguments for surgical and non-surgical treatment are balanced.

4.1.2 Radicular Symptoms

4.1.2.1 Radicular Pain Syndrome

An acute disc herniation with compression of ventral and dorsal spinal nerve roots causes a radicular pain syndrome that not just affects the dermatome but also the sclerotome. In cases of the more frequent, slowly progressive spondylosis, the pain syndrome begins with a dull and gnawing pain in the neck and shoulder followed by the arm. Later paraesthesias and a sensation of numbness appear. Some patients suffer from sudden fulgurous pain that can be triggered by moving the head or coughing (Frykholm 1969).

The deep somatic pain which is often described as dull pain results from compression of the ventral root. Neuralgia with paraesthesias and numbness that radiates into fingers is the result of dorsal nerve root compression (Frykholm 1969).

4.1.2.2 Sensory Deficits

Disorders of sensation usually start distally at the fingers. There it is easy to identify the border of the affected dermatome and thus the compressed nerve root. Paraesthesias are a symptom of intermittent compression of the dorsal nerve root. They can appear in combination with hypoalgesia or hyperalgesia (Frykholm 1969). A reduced sensation of vibration (pallhypaesthesia) is considered as a sign of multiradicular compression and is mainly used to detect differential diagnoses such as polyneuropathy.

4.1.2.3 Motor Deficits

The compression of a ventral root causes paresis of a segment-indicating muscle and in some cases atrophy of muscles. Pareses with high functional consequences and acute severe motor deficits, respectively, are main indicators for surgical treatment in cases of proven cervical disc herniation. The clinical identification of nerve root compression reliably succeeds in cases of weakness of a segment-indicating muscle (O'Brien 2000):

- C4: major and minor rhomboideus muscle
- C5: deltoid muscle

- C6: biceps and brachioradialis muscles
- C7: triceps muscle
- C8: superficial flexor digitorum, deep flexor digitorum I and II, deep flexor digitorum III and IV muscles
- T1: opponens pollicis muscle and muscles of the hypothenar

4.1.2.4 Vegetative Disorders

Some patients with nerve root compression suffer from an increased tone of the sympathetic nervous system with consecutive vasomotoric disorders of the upper limb leading to a sensation of coldness and a change of skin colour. A cervicocephal syndrome was described by Barré (1926). It is characterised by unilateral headaches, vertigo, sometimes tinnitus and ear pain.

4.1.3 Pathological Reflexes as a Sign of Radicular or Spinal Cord Compression

The monosynaptic muscle reflexes are diminished in cases of compression of a peripheral nerve such as hyporeflexia of the triceps reflex as a sign of compression of the C7 root. Hyperreflexia (a response far larger than considered normal) can be seen if there is a lack of central nervous inhibitory signals, e.g. very brisk response of the patellar reflex due to compression of the cervical spinal cord as a reason of disorder of the pyramidal tracts.

The polysynaptic reflexes can be reduced in cases of pyramidal tract lesions, for example, an absent abdominal reflex as a consequence of spinal cord compression due to a cervical spondylotic myelopathy.

Reduced or absent reflexes of the upper limbs can be observed in case of a cervical disc herniation (affected nerve root in brackets):

- Biceps reflex (C6)
- Brachioradialis reflex (C5, C6)
- Triceps reflex (C7)
- Trömner's reflex (C7, C8)

Cervical spondylotic myelopathy often causes hyperactive patellar and Achilles tendon reflexes at the lower limbs as a sign of pyramidal tract disorder. Furthermore, a positive Babinski sign is noticed that is also a typical sign of pyramidal tract disorder.

4.1.4 Myelopathic Symptoms: Spondylotic Myelopathy

Spinal cord compression of a higher grade during degenerative diseases of the cervical spine often appears as chronic state in case of an osteoligamentous spinal stenosis. MR images often show a so-called myelopathy signal as a typical finding.

This signal appears in sagittal T2-weighted images as an intramedullary hyperintense area caudal to the stenosis (Fig. 4.3). Typical clinical findings are hyperreflexia of the lower limbs (Sect. 4.1.3), positive Babinski sign, unstableness in coordination tests (Unterberger's stepping test, tightrope walking test, etc.), increased tone of lower limb muscles, sustained cloni at the lower limbs, pallhypaesthesia, fine motor disorders and non-radicular loss of sensation on both hands. In rare cases patients also suffer from centrally caused vegetative disorders such as bladder and bowel incontinence.

In the rare case of acute massive cervical disc herniation, a paraplegia can be observed with a positive Lhermitte sign. This can be triggered by passive flection of the cervical spine and leads to a sensation of needles and pins.

4.2 Imaging

4.2.1 Magnetic Resonance Imaging (MRI)

If cervical radiculopathy or myelopathy is clinically suspicious for a cervical disc herniation, then MRI is the imaging modality of first choice because it excellently visualises ligaments, discs and neural structures (Figs. 6.2 and 6.3). If so also other pathologies causing such symptoms can be identified (e.g. tumours or inflammations).

Typical MRI findings are:

- Soft disc herniation (Fig. 4.1): acute or subacute herniation, more often seen in younger patients
- Hard disc herniation (Fig. 4.2): chronified herniation with loss of fluid within the disc and transition to an osteoligamentous stenosis, more often seen in elderly patients
- Osteoligamentous spinal stenosis with myelopathic signal in sagittal T2-weighted images caudal to the stenosis (Fig. 4.3)

4.2.2 Computed Tomography (CT)

Computed tomography is able to deliver useful additional information for the planning of surgical strategy in cases of significant dorsal osteophytes at the vertebral body or pathological ossification of the posterior longitudinal ligament (Fig. 4.4) since osteophytes are best visualised in the so-called bone window of a CT scan. Furthermore, a CT imaging is useful in cases of diffuse idiopathic skeletal hyperostosis (Fig. 4.5).

After anterior plating and/or posterior instrumentation of the cervical spine, a CT scan is crucial to document the right position of the implants (Figs. 4.4b and 4.5d).

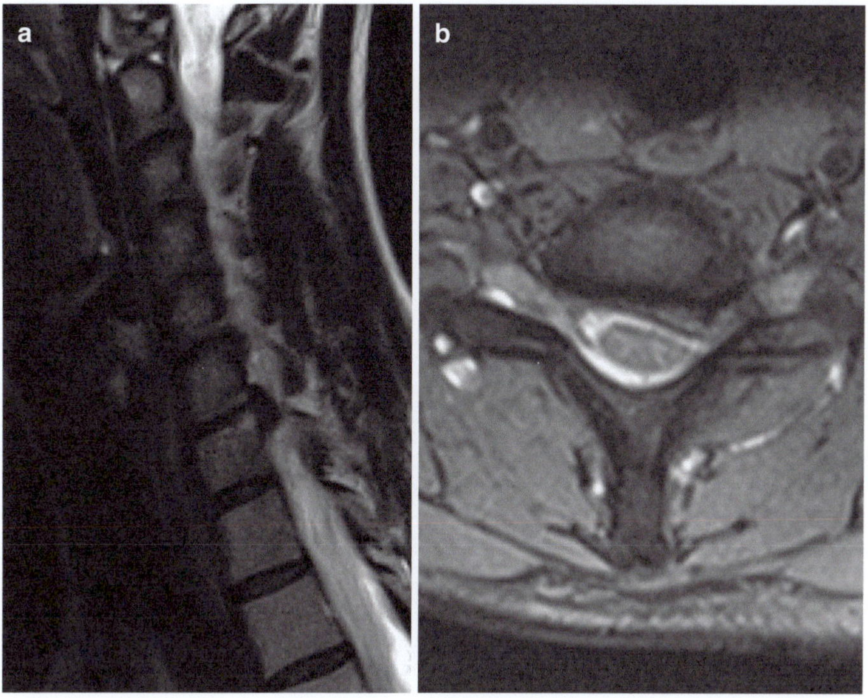

Fig. 4.1 Soft disc herniation at the C6/C7 level on the left side, sagittal (**a**) and axial (**b**) T2-weighted MR images

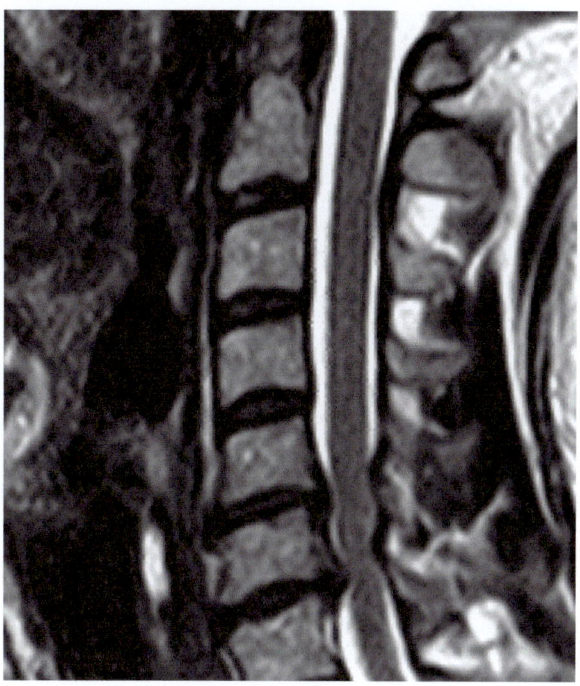

Fig. 4.2 Hard disc herniation at the C5/C6 and C6/C7 levels, sagittal T2-weighted MR image

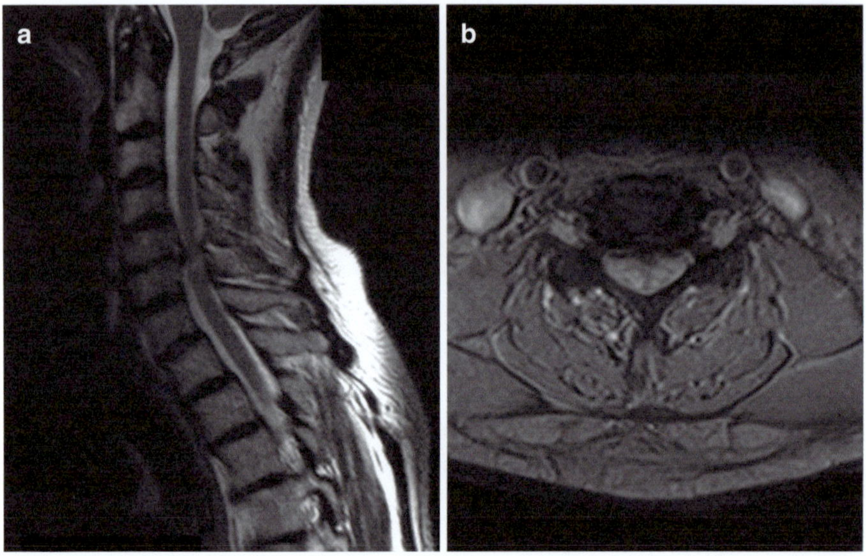

Fig. 4.3 Osteoligamentous spinal stenosis with chronic myelopathy at the level C5/C6. Sagittal (**a**) and axial (**b**) T2-weighted MR images. It is clearly to be seen that the myelopathic signal is located caudal to the narrowed level in the sagittal slices. In the axial image, it can be seen that the myelopathic signal is predominantly located in the posterior aspect of the spinal cord

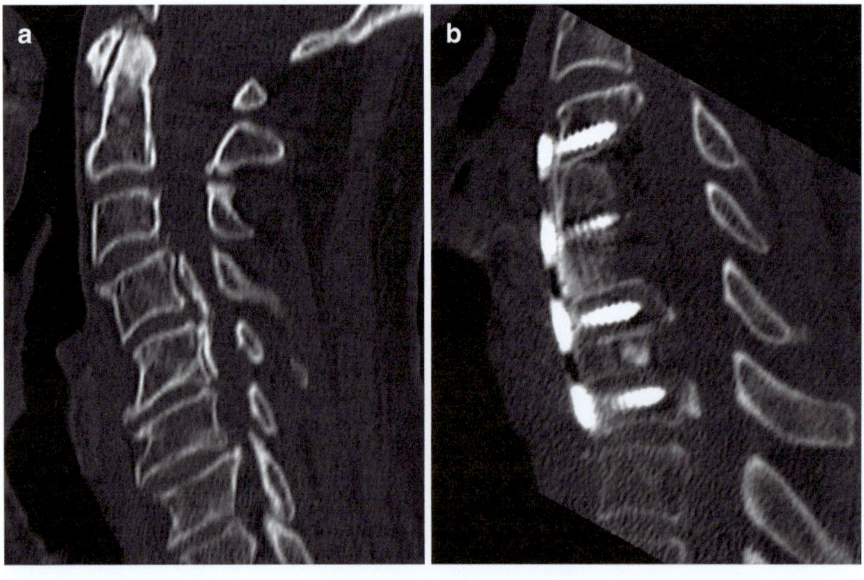

Fig. 4.4 Ossification of the posterior longitudinal ligament at the posterior vertebral bodies of C4 and C5 as well as posterior osteophytes and the C6/C7 level, sagittal CT in the bone window (**a**). Situation after corpectomy of C4 and C5 with resection of the posterior longitudinal ligament as well as after discectomy at C6/C7 with resection of osteophytes. Furthermore, interposition of an iliac crest bone graft between C3 and C6 as well as cage implantation at C6/C7 and anterior plating from C3 to C7, sagittal CT in the bone window (**b**)

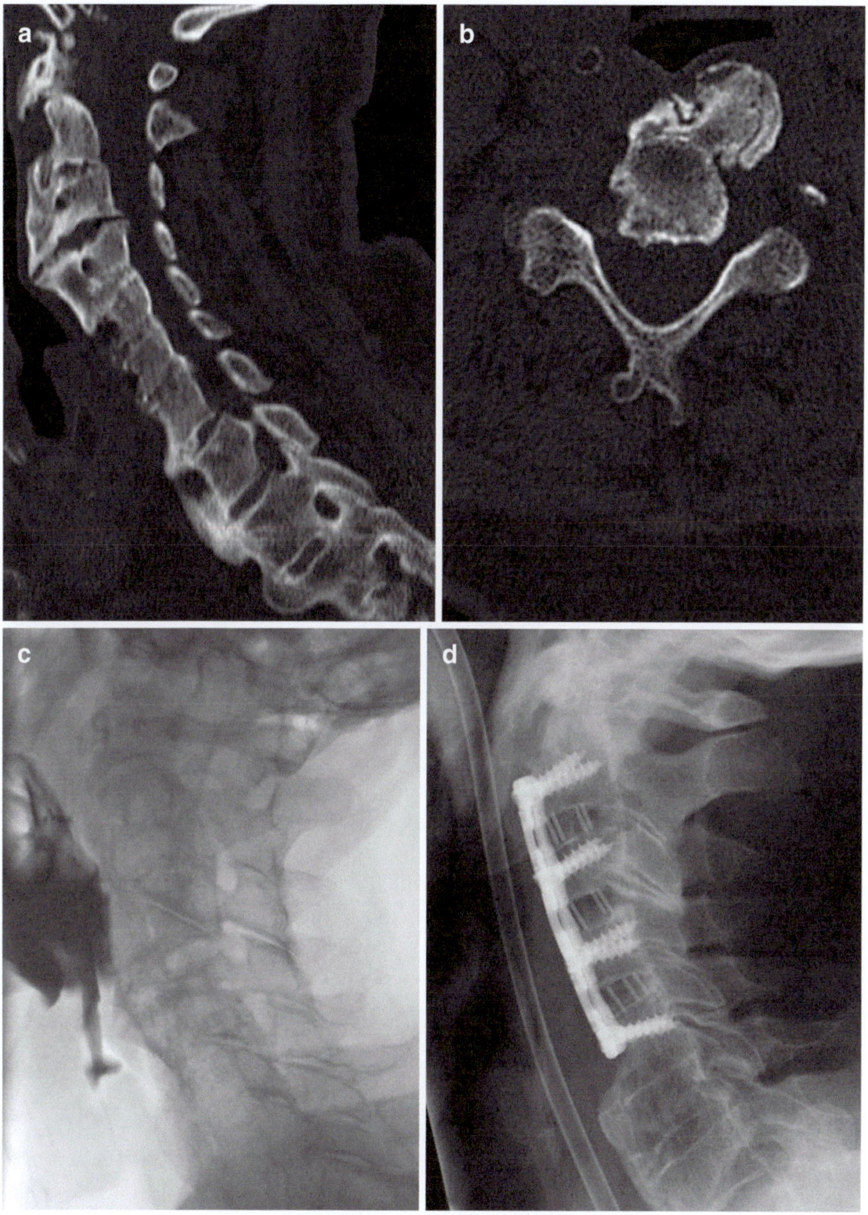

Fig. 4.5 Diffuse idiopathic skeletal hyperostosis with typical giant osteophytes at the whole cervical spine and consecutive dysphagia, sagittal (**a**) and axial (**b**) CT images as well as barium swallow X-ray (**c**). Status after resection of the ventral osteophytes and anterior plating to avoid recurrence of the osteophytes, lateral X-ray examination (**d**)

4.2.3 X-Ray

Conventional X-ray imaging of the cervical spine in two planes shows ventral osteophytes, facet joint arthrosis and kyphotic or scoliotic malposition of vertebral bodies.

Due to the progressive widespread of cervical prostheses for total disc replacement, the significance of lateral functional X-ray images has emerged because motility of the affected level as well as of the adjacent levels can be assessed (Figs. 7.3, 7.4 and 7.5). Basically, it is also possible to take anterior-posterior X-ray images but these are not of high significance in clinical practice since lateral bending is not as important as flexion/extension of the cervical spine.

Recently, reference objects are used in functional imaging to enable computerised analysis of the range of motion and thus to increase the measurement accuracy and the comparability of segmental motion in functional X-rays before and after total disc replacement (Fig. 4.6).

Barium swallow X-ray images show in cases of diffuse idiopathic skeletal hyperostosis and consecutive dysphagia the maximum of the oesophageal stenosis (Fig. 4.5c). Furthermore, they are of diagnostic value after dislocation of anterior osteosynthesis material (Fig. 4.7).

4.2.4 Myelography and Myelo-CT

Due to the combination of MRI, CT and X-ray imaging, the significance of cervical myelography has decreased although for safety reasons the application of the contrast agent is done in the lumbar and not in the suboccipital region.

Myelography and myelo-CT can be useful in cases of multilevel disease (Fig. 4.8) or after previous surgery with implants (Fig. 4.9) since in the latter case, MRI often produces artefacts and thus neural structures cannot be visualised.

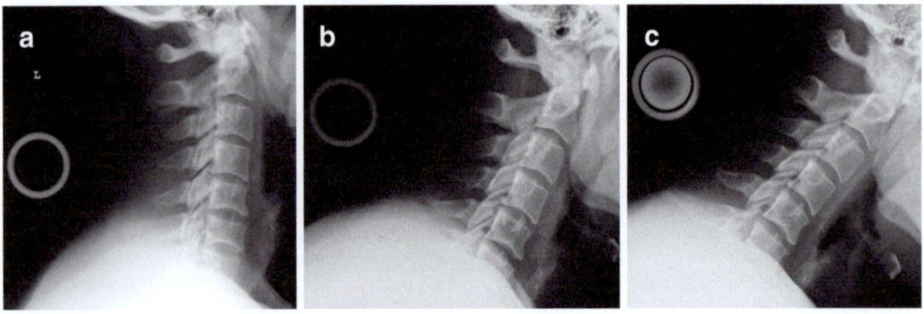

Fig. 4.6 Lateral functional X-ray images with reference object for computer-aided analysis of segmental range of motion in extension (**a**), neutral position (**b**) and flexion (**c**)

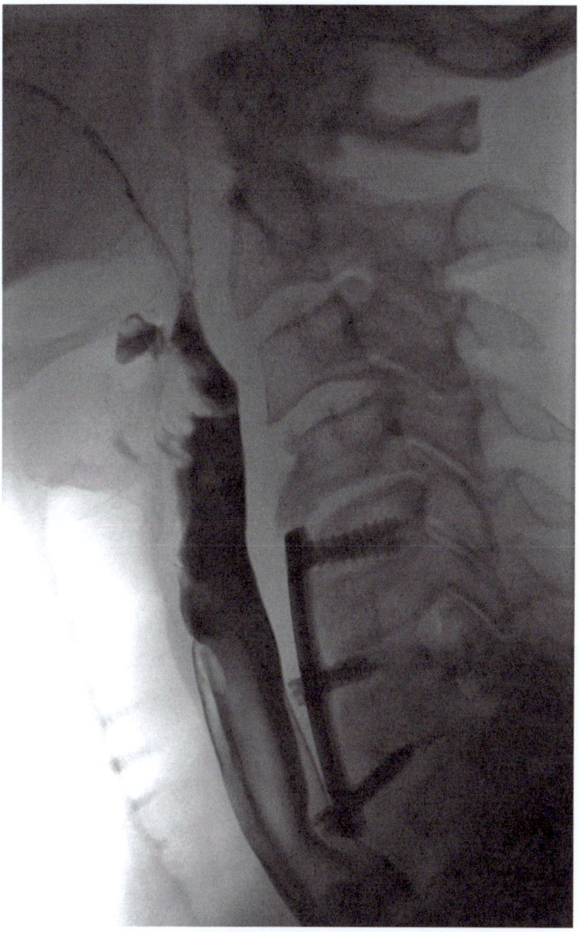

Fig. 4.7 Barium swallow X-ray to verify impingement of the oesophagus in a patient with dysphagia due to a dislocated anterior plate after loosening of screws in the lowest vertebral body of the osteosynthesis. Thus, there is an indication for revision surgery

4.2.5 Image-Guided Nerve Root and Facet Joint Infiltration

If there is clinical insecurity about the compression of a certain nerve root, it is possible to reduce the pain and identify the affected nerve root with the help of CT-guided nerve root infiltration, especially in cases of multilevel stenosis of the neural foramina (Fig. 4.10). Analogue to this, it is possible to reduce neck pain without radicular pain by performing an image-guided facet joint infiltration, whereas at the cervical spine, CT guidance is mainly used because of its higher accuracy (Fig. 4.11).

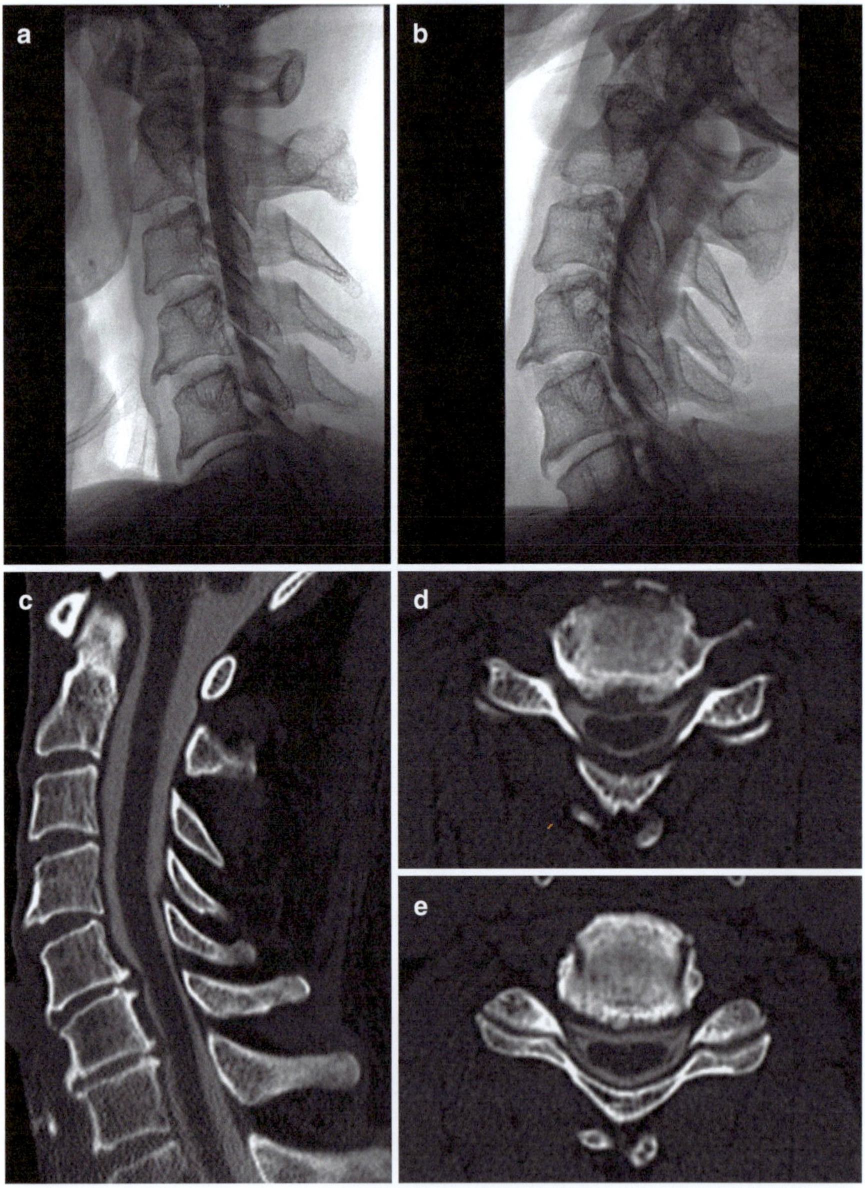

Fig. 4.8 Cervical myelography, lateral images in flexion (**a**) and extension (**b**). Sagittal myelo-CT showing an osteochondrosis at C5/C6 and C6/C7 (**c**). Axial myelo-CT with demonstration of the osteochondrosis at C5/C6 (**d**) and the intradural course of the anterior and posterior C6 roots (**e**)

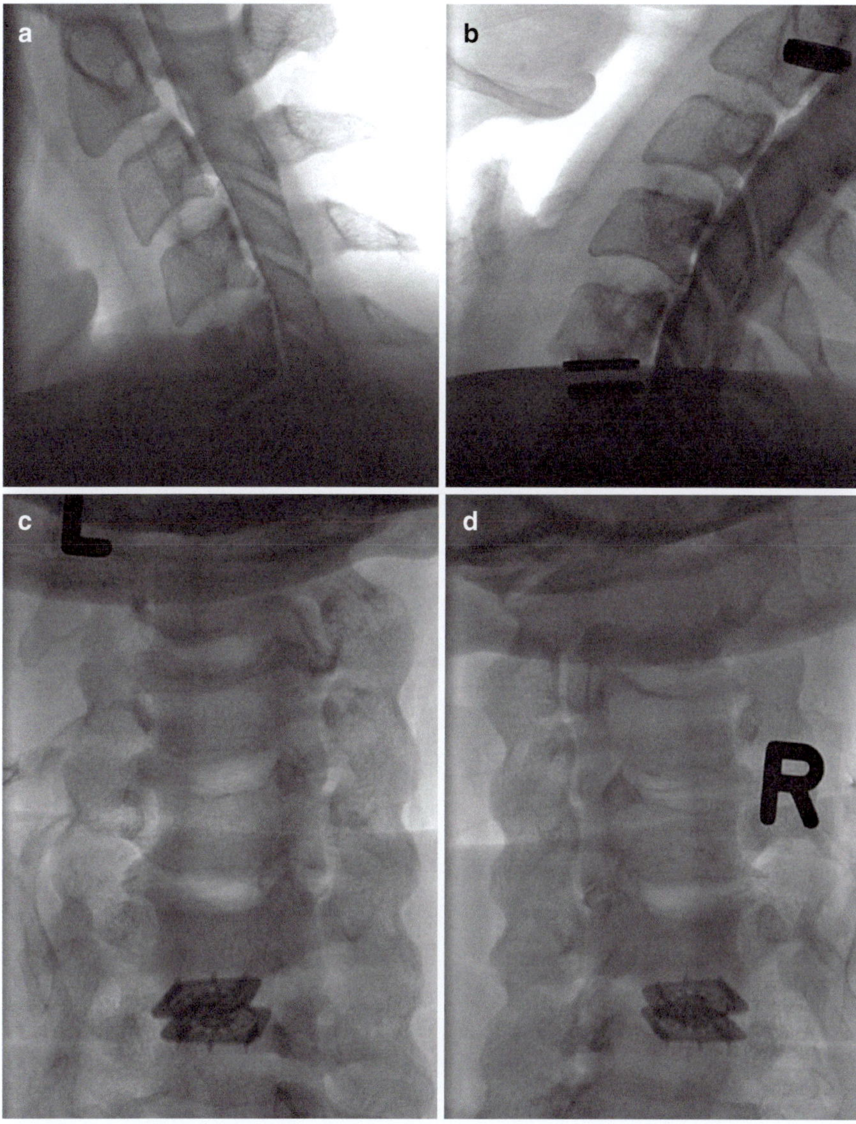

Fig. 4.9 Cervical functional myelography after total disc replacement with an M6C prosthesis at C5/C6, lateral images in flexion (**a**) and extension (**b**) as well as oblique anterior-posterior images showing the proximal nerve roots at the left (**c**) and right (**d**). There are no signs of compression of neural structures at the operated level

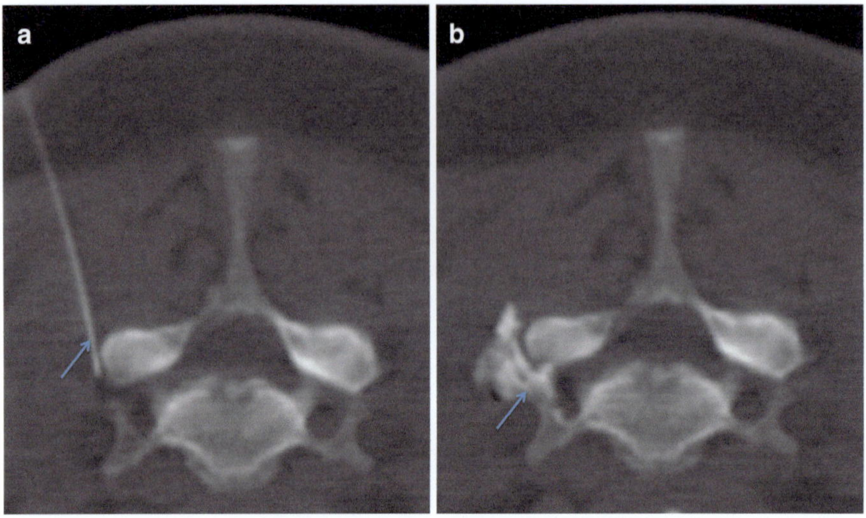

Fig. 4.10 CT-guided nerve root infiltration with local anaesthetics of the left C7 root for differential diagnosis. Axial CT image showing the injection needle (**a**) and final application of contrast agent to document the infiltration (**b**)

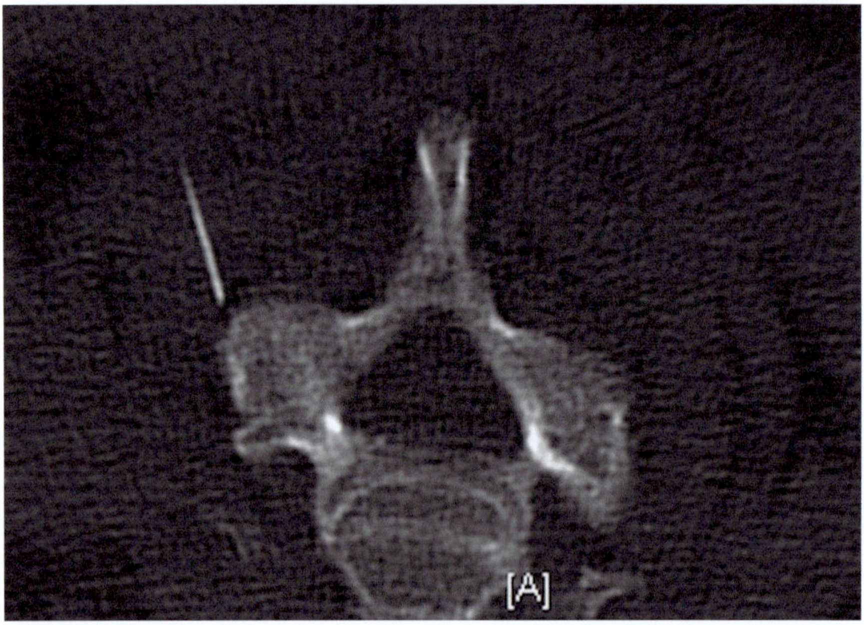

Fig. 4.11 CT-guided facet joint infiltration at C5/C6 on the left side

This advantage of computed tomography is accompanied by the disadvantage of a higher exposure to radiation compared to X-ray imaging, but finally the advantages outweigh the disadvantages especially in the lower cervical levels C6/C7 and C7/T1 where adequate X-ray visualisation is often difficult due to the shoulders.

The nerve root infiltration as well as the facet joint infiltration is done with a local anaesthetic. If the infiltration leads to significant pain relief and if there is no indication for surgery due to a lack of morphological findings, then the procedure can be repeated with an additional steroid (usually triamcinolone). It is supposed that an additional steroid leads to long-lasting pain relief due to its anti-inflammatory effect and detumescence. Thus, nerve root infiltration can be considered as semi-causal treatment.

4.3 Electrophysiology

In cases of degenerative diseases of the cervical spine, electrophysiological examinations can be a useful supplement of clinical and radiological findings, especially in the following situations (Bischoff and Schulte-Mattler 2011):

- Identifying the mainly affected nerve root in cases of multiradicular symptoms
- Differentiating between radicular and peripheral nerve symptoms, e.g. C6 or C7 syndrome versus carpal tunnel syndrome
- Estimation of the severity of cervical spondylotic myelopathy by the use of somatosensory evoked potentials in cases of mismatch between clinical and radiological findings

For example, a carpal tunnel syndrome is unlikely if the distal motor latency and the distal motor nerve conduction study of the median nerve as well as the electromyogram (EMG) of the abductor pollicis brevis muscle are normal. If there are signs of axonal injury in the EMGs of the muscles being innervated by C6 and C7, the patient probably suffers from radicular symptoms (Milnik 2012).

References

Barré JA. Le syndrome sympathique cervical postérieur. Rev Neurol. 1926;33:248–9.

Bischoff C, Schulte-Mattler WJ. Das EMG-Buch. Stuttgart: Thieme; 2011.

Frykholm R. Die cervicalen Bandscheibenschäden. In: Olivecrona H, Tönnis W (Hrsg.) Handbuch der Neurochirurgie. Siebenter Band/Erster Teil. Berlin/Heidelberg/New York: Springer; 1969.

Milnik V. Elektrophysiologie in der Praxis. München: Elsevier; 2012.

O'Brien MD. Aids to the examination of the peripheral nervous system. Edinburgh/London/New York/Oxford: Elsevier Saunders; 2000.

5 Conservative Treatment

Conservative treatment in cases of degenerative diseases of the cervical spine primarily addresses pain relief. For this nonsteroidal anti-inflammatory drugs (NSAID) and, where required, additional central analgesics are applied. Physiotherapy focuses on passive procedures in the acute phase. In the subacute and rehab phase (after surgery or also for conservative cases), active exercises are added. Physical therapeutical methods are massages, application of warmth or cold and electrotherapy. Psychotherapy can be indicated in cases of chronic complaints with the absence of morphological findings in imaging.

5.1 General Considerations

If a patient is suffering from short-term neck-shoulder-arm pain without or slight neurological deficits, a conservative treatment for 6–8 weeks is indicated. Furthermore, conservative treatment is indicated for patients with chronic complaints but without pathological findings in the MR imaging. During conservative therapy the patient must be informed about the possibility of progressive motor deficits and the necessity of urgent readmission to the hospital and the indication for surgery in this case.

Conservative treatment includes multimodal analgetic therapy and physiotherapy as well as psychotherapy in selected cases with psychosomatic or chronified complaints. The primary goal of conservative treatment is pain relief, especially in the acute phase. Therefore, during physiotherapy the focus is on procedures with pain relief potential such as massage, traction, manual therapeutical procedures, application of warmth or cold and electrotherapy (Sect. 5.3). In the subacute and rehab phase, treatment is more focused on active physiotherapy to achieve muscular stabilisation of the spine.

A. König, U. Spetzger, *Degenerative Diseases of the Cervical Spine*,
DOI 10.1007/978-3-319-47298-0_5

The best prognosis for a success of conservative treatment can be expected in cases of soft disc herniation since pain causing nerve root compression can regress because of the morphological finding.

5.2 Pain Management

5.2.1 Nonsteroidal Anti-inflammatory Drugs (NSAIDs)

NSAIDs are the medication of first choice for the symptomatic treatment of pain due to degenerative diseases of the spine. Their principle of operation is an inhibition of cyclooxygenase (prostaglandin-endoperoxide synthase) in the prostaglandin metabolism (Kellner 2005). The mainly used classical NSAIDs are diclofenac and ibuprofen.

Diclofenac is a derivate of aryl acetic acid and has anti-inflammatory, analgetic and antipyretic effects. The plasma half-life is 1–2 h. The elimination is mainly renal (Offermanns 2012).

Ibuprofen is a derivate of aryl propionic acid and has similar effects as diclofenac. The plasma half-life is about 2 h (Offermanns 2012).

In cases of longer application, it is indicated to combine the NSAIDs with a proton-pump inhibitor (e.g. pantoprazole) to avoid gastrointestinal side effects.

Besides the systemic application, it might be useful to applicate NSAIDs locally for the treatment of neck pain.

The WHO suggests a three-step analgesic ladder for medicamentous pain management, whereas step 1 (mild pain) includes the application of NSAIDs only (Diener 2005). For moderate pain (step 2), the application of an NSAID and/or paracetamol in combination with a weak opioid such as tramadol is recommended. Severe pain (step 3) requires the combination of an NSAID and/or paracetamol with a strong opioid (Table. 5.1).

5.2.2 Central Analgetics

If the application of an NSAID only is not effective for pain management, then the addition of a central analgetic should be considered. According to the WHO analgesic ladder, the mainly used drug in clinical practice is the opioid tramadol. For the treatment of spinal caused pain, it can be combined with metamizole and dexamethasone (optional) and applied intravenously. With this medication it is usually possible to manage even severe neck and arm pain due to cervical disc herniation.

Table 5.1 Stepwise scheme of pain management as recommended by the WHO (Diener 2005)

Step	Pharmaceutical drug	Examples
1	Non-opioid analgetics	NSAID, Metamizole, Paracetamol
2	Non-opioid analgetics and weak opioids	Tramadol, Tilidine
3	Non opioid analgetics and strong opioids	Morphine, Oxycodone, Fentanyl

Patients with chronic pain and without a surgical option can be treated with a transdermal opioid patch. A multimodal pain management in chronified cases should be initiated by a specialised pain therapist.

5.3 Physiotherapy

5.3.1 Aim of Treatment and Instruction of the Patient

A main principle of physiotherapy is instructing the patient how motional behaviour in the daily life can be improved to avoid inappropriate biomechanical stresses. Besides instructions there should be controls and corrections on a regular basis. By doing so the patient learns self-help strategies to avoid pain and increase his or her effectiveness. Another step is the instruction of the patient for independent exercising at home. The number and complexity of the exercises should be moderate to achieve an adequate compliance.

An example is the suboccipital self-massage of muscles. In this exercise the patient supports his head in sitting position and massages the suboccipital muscles with the other hand. Due to the self-massage of muscles, the patient trains self-perception (Wiesner 2012).

5.3.2 Motion Therapy

In the state of acute neck and arm pain, motion therapy is not indicated but pain relief is the most important aim of treatment.

In the subacute phase and during rehabilitation after surgery, active elements like isometric tension exercises or complex motion exercises with good axial alignment can strengthen the neck muscles. If a cervical disc herniation leads to weakness of a certain muscle of the upper limb due to compression of a motor nerve root, it is crucial to train especially this muscle since dysfunction of arm or hand muscles has significant functional consequences.

Patients with cervical spondylotic myelopathy often suffer from coordination disorders of the lower limbs; thus, special gait training during rehabilitation is necessary.

Further physiotherapeutical methods are mobilisation, extension and traction (Papathanasiou 2012).

5.3.3 Vojta Method (Reflex Locomotion)

This treatment was established in the 1960s by Czech neurologist Václav Vojta as a physiotherapy for disorders of the central nervous system and the musculoskeletal system. Its principle is based on the reactivation of physiological patterns of motion in patients with neurologically triggered motion disorders or orthopaedic posture abnormalities (Vojta 2007). Primarily the Vojta method was established for the treatment of infants and children; nowadays it is also used in the rehabilitation of adults. During treatment pressure is applied to a certain body zone in a defined position whereby reflex motion patterns are involuntary triggered. By adapting the trigger zones, the treatment is tuned to the patient's aim of therapy.

5.3.4 Massage

Patients with degenerative diseases of the cervical spine often describe a positive short-term effect after massage (local pain relief). Despite the short-term effect of the massage, it is reasonable to repeatedly interrupt the circuit of abnormal muscle tension and neck pain. Myogeloses (local increase of muscle tension) are a typical indication for a classical massage treatment.

Massage of neck muscles usually includes a massage of the whole back since the autochthonous and allochthonous muscles of the back make up a complex system that works as a whole.

The massage usually starts with flat strokes that are combined with circulating strokes, oblique strokes, hand-over-hand strokes and the rake grasp. The latter is a combination of moving knuckles upwards and friction downwards with fingertips. Depending on palpation findings, frictions, fascia strokes or skin techniques can be included (Junker 2007). Specific treatments of the cervical region are circular strokes of neck muscles, oblique kneading of the trapezius muscle and frictions of the supraspinatus muscle (Kolster 2010).

5.3.5 Cryotherapy and Thermotherapy

The primary goal of cryotherapy or thermotherapy in the treatment of degenerative diseases of the cervical spine is pain relief. Their effects have to be tested individually for each patient. During extensive thermotherapy in elderly patients, special emphasis has to be put on cardiovascular events.

Cold is usually applied as repeated short baths (few seconds up to 1 min) with a water temperature below 20 °C (Uehleke 2012). The therapeutic principle of pain relief is based on reactive hyperaemia after the application of the cold.

A possible kind of thermotherapy is the application of peloid packs with a temperature of 45–50 °C on the back. The application time is about 30 min. It could be shown that a biomechanical effect of peloids is an inhibition of prostaglandin and leukotriene synthesis (Uehleke 2012) that finally leads to pain relief. The application of vasodilatative ointments also has an analgetic effect and generates a sensation of warmth.

5.3.6 Electrotherapy

The most frequently used method of electrotherapeutical techniques for the treatment of neck pain and myogeloses is the transcutaneous electrical nerve stimulation (TENS). It can be done by a therapist or a patient himself or herself

(Junker 2007). The patient's pain coping can be improved by this active engagement with complaints.

There are different empirical setups for the placement of electrodes and kind of impulse for the different types of spondylotic pain (Hankemeier and Krizanits-Weine 2010). Diffuse spondylotic pain without radicular symptoms responses well to co-current flow impulses with a frequency of 30–150 Hz. The electrodes for stimulation are placed paravertebral cranial and caudal to the area of pain.

The paraesthesias triggered by TENS cover the back pain during therapy. Radicular pain is also treated with pulses of 30–150 Hz. The cathode is placed next to the spine, and the anode is placed distally. The stimulus is supposed to cover the pain. As an alternative a low-frequency stimulation with 0.5–5 Hz in burst mode can be applied. The anode is placed next to the spine, and the cathode is placed peripheral. This method triggers muscle contractions that cause pain relief proportional to their intensity. Pseudoradicular pain is treated with high-frequency stimulation above the causing structure, whereas the paravertebral muscles should not show contraction under stimulation (Hankemeier and Krizantis-Weine 2010).

Thus, TENS is an interface between physical therapy and pain management since after successful TENS analgetics can be reduced (Bezerra et al. 2011).

5.4 Psychotherapy

Psychotherapy for the treatment of neck or back pain can be indicated in two different situations:

in patients with clinical complaints but without morphological findings of nerve root compression in MR imaging, psychosomatic reasons for the pain have to be ruled out or treated, especially if psychosocial factors are maintaining conditions for the pain (Kröner-Herwig 2011).

Furthermore, patients with chronic pain and resistance to conservative and surgical therapy require an adequate psychotherapeutic treatment because the state of chronic pain can lead to a narrowing of life perspective and resignation.

Important risk factors for a chronified course of disease are:

- Fixed ideas about the course of treatment
- Increased attention to physical symptoms
- Abuse of medication
- Overprotective partner
- Dissatisfaction at work
- Belief that only somatic treatment is effective
- Dissatisfaction about previous treatment (Pfingsten and Hildebrandt 2011)

A possible therapeutic approach is cognitive behavioural therapy. Initially, a situation analysis identifies stress factors and pain-triggering situations, and the patient's patterns of behaviour are analysed. Afterwards aims of changes and feasible steps for reaching these aims have to be defined (Pfingsten et al. 2011). An alternative method is depth psychologically founded psychotherapy where the focus is on analysing unconscious or suppressed conflicts in the past.

References

Bezerra P, Zhou S, Crowley Z, et al. Effects of electromyostimulation on knee extensors and flexors strength and steadiness in older adults. J Mot Beahv. 2011;43(5):413–21.

Diener HC. Neurologische Erkrankungen. In: Wehling M (Hrsg) Klinische Pharmakologie. Stuttgart: Thieme; 2005.

Hankemeier UB, Krizanits-Weine FH. Vertebragene Schmerzen. In: Pothmann R (Hrsg) TENS: Transkutane elektrische Nervenstimulation in der Schmerztherapie. Stuttgart: Hippokrates; 2010. p. S34–38.

Junker HO. Massage. In: Hüter-Becker A, Dölken M (Hrsg) Physikalische Therapie, Massage, Elektrotherapie und Lymphdrainage. Stuttgart: Thieme; 2007.

Kellner H. Entzündlich-rheumatische Erkrankungen. In: Wehling M (Hrsg) Klinische Pharmakologie. Stuttgart: Thieme; 2005.

Kolster BC. Massage: Klassische Massage, Querfriktionen, Funktionsmassage. Heidelberg/Berlin: Springer; 2010.

Kröner-Herwig B. Schmerz als biopsychosoziales Phänomen – eine Einführung. In: Kröner-Herwig B, Frettlöh J, Klinger R, Nilges P (Hrsg) Schmerzpsychotherapie: Grundlagen – Diagnostik – Krankheitsbilder – Behandlung. Berlin/Heidelberg: Springer; 2011.

Offermanns S. Antiphlogistika und Antiallergika. In: Freissmuth M, Offermanns S, Böhm S (Hrsg) Pharmakologie und Toxikologie: Von den molekularen Grundlagen zur Pharmakotherapie. Heidelberg: Springer Medizin; 2012.

Papathanasiu A, Schüle K. Krankengymnastik (Physiotherapie). In: Beer AM, Adler M (Hrsg) Leitfaden Naturheilverfahren für die ärztliche Praxis. München: Urban und Fischer; 2012.

Pfingsten M, Hildebrandt J. Rückenschmerzen. In: Kröner-Herwig B, Frettlöh J, Klinger R, et al. (Hrsg) Schmerzpsychotherapie: Grundlagen – Diagnostik – Krankheitsbilder – Behandlung. Berlin/Heidelberg: Springer; 2011.

Pfingsten M, Korb J, Hasenbring M. Psychologische Mechanismen der Chronifizierung – Konsequenzen für die Prävention. In: Kröner-Herwig B Frettlöh J, Klinger R, et al. (Hrsg) Schmerzpsychotherapie: Grundlagen – Diagnostik – Krankheitsbilder – Behandlung. Berlin/Heidelberg: Springer; 2011.

Uehleke B. Bädertherapie. In: Beer AM, Adler M (Hrsg) Leitfaden Naturheilverfahren für die ärztliche Praxis. München: Urban und Fischer; 2012.

Vojta V, Peters A. Das Vojta-Prinzip: Muskelspiele in Reflexfortbewegung und motorischer Ontogenese. Berlin/Heidelberg: Springer; 2007.

Wiesner R. Übungen in der Physiotherapie. Stuttgart: Thieme; 2012.

6 Choice of Surgical Approach

In most cases of degenerative diseases of the cervical spine, the neural structures are compressed from anterior; thus, the anterior approach is the mainly used surgical approach to the cervical spine. The posterior approach is suitable for findings with ligamentous hypertrophy and space-occupying facet joint arthrosis as well as for elderly patients with spontaneous bony fusion in the intervertebral spaces where as lordosis is an essential precondition for this approach. Combined approaches are indicated in cases of corpectomy of two or more vertebral bodies and generally in cases with reduced bone quality due to a metabolic diseases such as osteoporosis, diabetes mellitus or renal failure.

6.1 Anterior Approach

Anterior cervical discectomy and fusion (ACDF) is the most commonly used procedure for the surgical treatment of cervical spondylotic radiculopathy and myelopathy since most space-occupying structures originate from intervertebral discs, posterior longitudinal ligament and vertebral bodies and thus are located anteriorly to the spinal cord. A corpectomy is indicated in cases of a confluent multilevel stenosis because this kind of stenosis continues from disc space to disc space behind the vertebral body (Medow 2006; König 2013). For the surgical technique, see Sects. 8.1 and 8.2.

Especially after corpectomy the re-establishment of sagittal balance and cervical lordosis is a further goal of surgery besides decompression of neural structures (Park 2012). This is achieved by choosing an adequate vertebral body replacement and bending the anterior plate prior to implantation (see Chap. 7). Hussain et al. (2013) could show in a finite element model that range of motion and load for discs and facet joints in adjacent levels is least after anterior fusion followed by posterior and combined fusion.

A. König, U. Spetzger, *Degenerative Diseases of the Cervical Spine*,
DOI 10.1007/978-3-319-47298-0_6

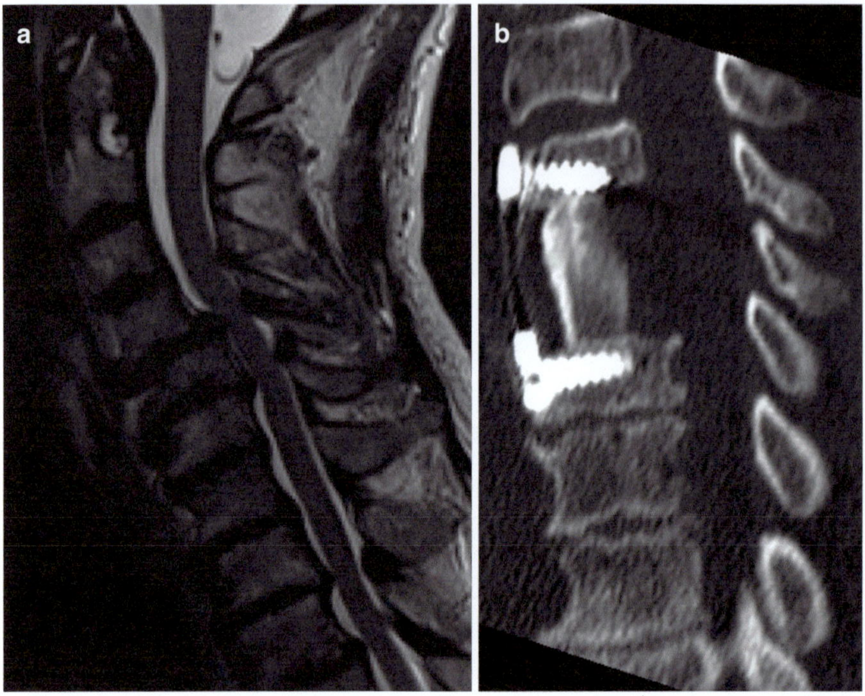

Fig. 6.1 Osteoligamentous spinal stenosis from C3 to C5 in a 66-year-old female, sagittal MRI (**a**). Corpectomy of C4 for decompression and vertebral body replacement with an iliac crest bone graft as well as anterior plating (system: Skyline, Synthes, Umkirch, Germany), sagittal CT scan (**b**)

These biomechanical stresses are considered as aetiological for accelerated adjacent level degeneration after fusion surgery (Kepler 2012). Thus, from a biomechanical point of view, the anterior approach for the surgical treatment of cervical radiculopathy and myelopathy should be preferred. This finding is of advantage for the clinical situation where most patients show space-occupying degenerative changes anterior to nerve roots and the spinal cord (Fig. 6.1).

6.2 Posterior Approach

For patients with predominant dorsal spinal cord compression, the surgeon can basically choose between two different procedures: laminectomy and lateral mass fusion (Fig. 6.2) or open-door laminoplasty (Fig. 6.3). For the surgical technique, see Sects. 8.3 and 8.4.

It could be shown that neurological outcome is the same for both procedures but laminectomy and fusion is associated with a significant reduction of neck pain compared to the open-door laminoplasty (Highsmith 2011).

The advantages of open-door laminoplasty are the maintenance of motion of the cervical spine, a reduced risk for morbidity due to screw malposition and,

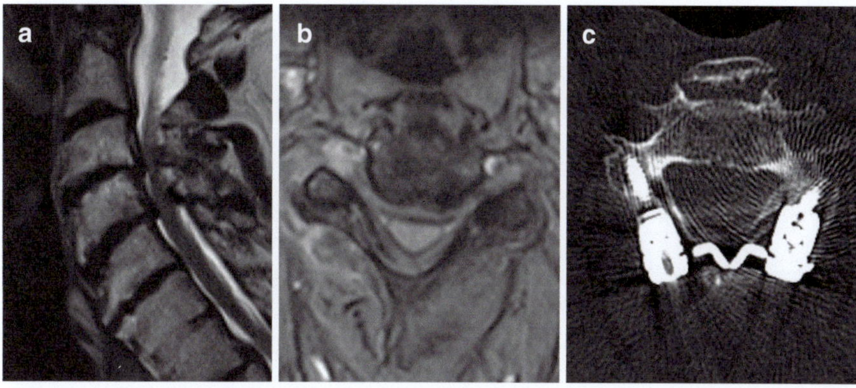

Fig. 6.2 Osteoligamentous spinal stenosis at levels C3/C4 and C4/C5 with predominant dorsal space occupation, sagittal (**a**) and axial MRI (**b**). Indication for posterior approach with decompression and fusion (system: Synapse, DePuy/Synthes), postoperative axial CT (**c**)

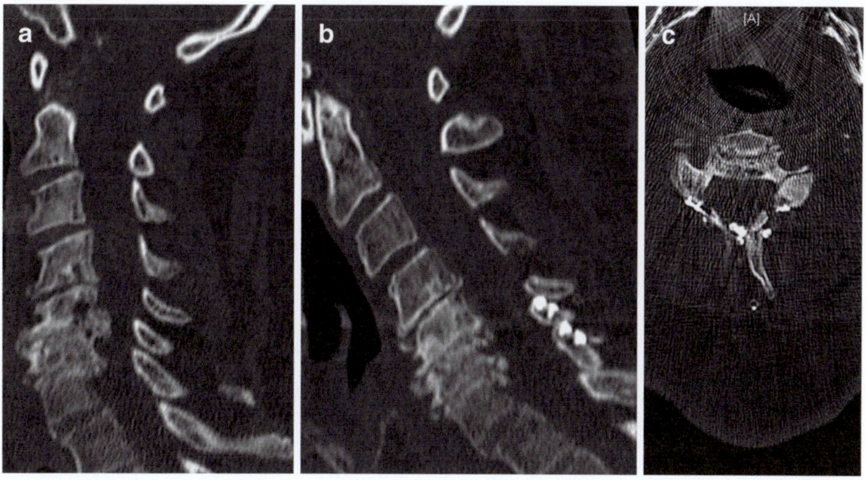

Fig. 6.3 CT scans of an 83-year-old patient with osteoligamentous spinal stenosis at levels C4/C5, C5/C6 and C6/C7, sagittal plane (**a**). The partial spontaneous bony fusion of vertebral bodies C5, C6 and C7 would make an anterior approach difficult. Therefore the spinal canal was widened by open-door laminoplasty, postoperative result in the sagittal (**b**) and axial plane (**c**)

especially in elderly patients with osteoporosis, a reduced risk for a breakout of the osteosynthesis.

Posterior procedures require a lordotic configuration of the cervical spine (Fig. 6.4). Fixed kyphotic abnormal postures are a contraindication for a posterior approach. In cases of significant osteoporosis with the risk of subsidence after vertebral body replacement, a posterior procedure can be better (Komotar 2006). A further indication for dorsal decompression is given if in elderly patients the intervertebral disc lost its height and the two adjacent vertebral bodies show spontaneous bony fusion.

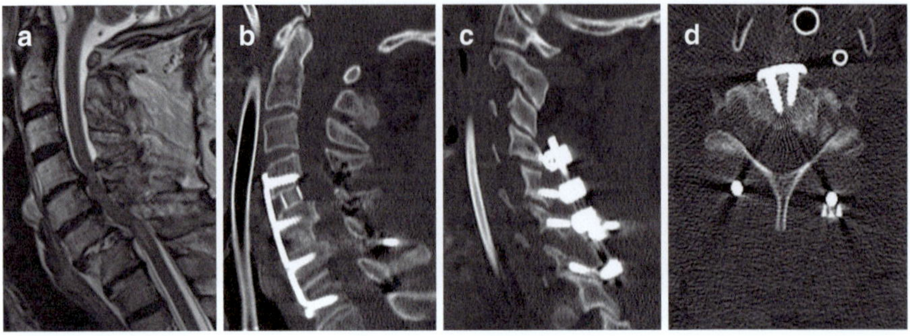

Fig. 6.4 Osteoligamentous spinal stenosis due to hard disc herniation at the levels C4/C5 and C5/C6 as well as traumatic instability at C6/C7, sagittal MRI (**a**). Sagittal (**b**, **c**) and axial (**d**) CT scan after combined approach and anterior-posterior stabilisation (systems: Skyline and Synapse)

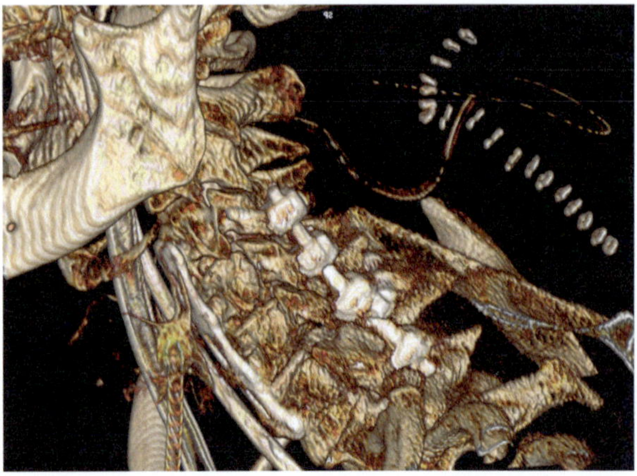

Fig. 6.5 Postoperative CT scan with 3D reconstruction of the same patient as in Fig. 6.4. Documentation of correct position of implants after anterior plating and posterior lateral mass fusion from C4 to C7

6.3 Combined Approach

For patients with significant kyphosis and/or proof of segmental instability (Figs. 6.4 and 6.5) due to degenerative changes, a combined approach with decompression and stabilisation is indicated, usually as a single-stage surgery.

Furthermore, a combined approach is indicated for patients with comorbidities that influence bone quality such as nicotine abuse, diabetes mellitus, rheumatoid arthritis or renal failure (Kim 2006; König 2013, 2014).

Since replacement of two or more vertebral bodies with anterior fusion only has an increased failure rate, it is recommended to add a posterior fusion in these cases (Kim 2006).

In general, combined multilevel instrumentations of the cervical spine have to be considered as surgeries with relatively high potential for surgical morbidities because the risks of anterior and posterior approach are added (see Chap. 10).

Possible complications might be a palsy of the laryngeal recurrent nerve with persisting hoarseness and dysphagia, life-threatening vascular complications or injury of the oesophagus and trachea with the potential risk of lethal mediastinitis. In cases of a breakout of implants, there might be no further surgical options except an external stabilisation with a halo vest. For those reason the indication for multi-level anterior-posterior surgical procedure has to be proven strictly.

References

Highsmith JM, Dhall SS, Haid RW, et al. Treatment of cervical stenotic myelopathy: a cost and outcome comparison of laminoplasty versus laminectomy and lateral mass fusion. J Neurosurg Spine. 2011;14(5):619–25.

Hussain M, Nassr A, Natarajan RN, et al. Biomechanics of adjacent segments after a multilevel cervical corpectomy using anterior, posterior, and combined anterior-posterior instrumentation techniques: a finite element model study. Spine J. 2013;13(6):689–96.

Kepler CK, Hilibrand AS. Management of adjacent segment disease after cervical spinal fusion. Orthop Clin North Am. 2012;43(1):53–62. viii

Kim PK, Alexander JT. Indications for circumferential surgery for cervical spondylotic myelopathy. Spine J. 2006;6(6 Suppl):299S–307S.

Komotar RJ, Mocco J, Kaiser MG. Surgical management of cervical myelopathy: indications and techniques for laminectomy and fusion. Spine J. 2006;6(6Suppl):252S–67S.

König SA, Ranguis S, Spetzger U. Management of complex cervical instability. J Neurol Surg A Cent Eur Neurosurg. 2013; doi:10.1055/s–0033–1345095.

König SA, Spetzger U. Surgical management of cervical spondylotic myelopathy – indications for anterior, posterior or combined procedures for decompression and stabilisation. Acta Neurochir. 2014;156(2):253–8.

Medow JE, Trost G, Sandin J. Surgical management of cervical myelopathy: indications and techniques for surgical corpectomy. Spine J. 2006;6(6 Suppl):233S–41S.

Park SB, Jahng TA, Chung CK. Remodeling of adjacent spinal alignments following cervical arthroplasty and anterior discectomy and fusion. Eur Spine J. 2012;21(2):322–7.

Choice of Implant

7

For younger patients with soft-disc herniation, only slight osteochondrosis, and good range of motion in the affected level the indication for total disc replacement with a cervical prosthesis is given. In elderly patients with hard-disc herniation, significant osteochondrosis, and reduced or absent range of motion in the affected level there is an indication for intervertebral cage fusion. For cervical vertebral body replacement, the use of autologous iliac crest bone graft is still the gold standard. Systems for anterior plating nowadays offer self-drilling screws and guiding instruments for correct screw angulation. Posterior fusion systems have become more user-friendly; thus, polyaxial screw heads make the insertion of connecting rods much easier. For open-door laminoplasty, it is possible to use microfixation systems from cranial surgery.

7.1 Disc Replacement

7.1.1 Total Disc Replacement: Prostheses

If a soft-disc herniation or osteoligamentous spinal stenosis at the level of the intervertebral disc is responsible for the patient's clinical symptoms, then neural structures can be adequately decompressed by doing a discectomy. After discectomy, the height of the intervertebral space has to be maintained to achieve an adequate height of the neuroforamina. Despite of that, it is remarkable that some departments in the 1980s did not use any implant but achieved clinical results that were comparable to other surgical methods (Bertalanffy and Eggert 1988).

Another aim of surgery, especially in younger patients, is the maintenance of motion in the affected level (Cardoso and Rosner 2010; Goel et al. 2012; Richards et al. 2012; Svedmark et al. 2011). Furthermore, the reestablishment of the

A. König, U. Spetzger, *Degenerative Diseases of the Cervical Spine*,
DOI 10.1007/978-3-319-47298-0_7

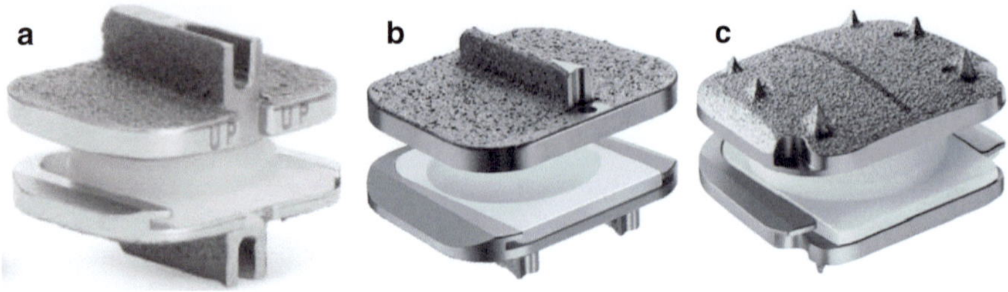

Fig. 7.1 Development of the anchor of cervical prostheses in the adjacent vertebral bodies: Prodisc-C with relatively big keels (**a**), Prodisc-C Nova with smaller keels (**b**) and Prodisc-C vivo with pins (**c**) (With kind permission from Synthes, Umkirch, Germany)

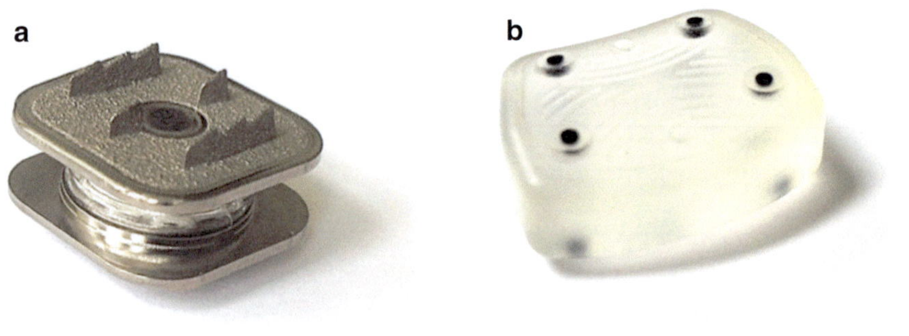

Fig. 7.2 Current cervical prostheses: Prosthesis M6C with plastic core and annulus as well as titanium endplates (**a**). Mono-block prosthesis Cadisc-C made of polyurethane (out of production since late 2015) (**b**)

physiological cervical lordosis after total disc replacement has become of interest for many spine surgeons (Bryan 2002; Le et al. 2004; Park et al. 2012). There is a general consensus about the fact that physiological motion at C2/3 and C7/T1 is relatively little and that it is not reasonable to implant a prosthesis (see Table 3.1). The level C3/4 is in an intermediate position – it is at the discretion of the surgeon to indicate total disc replacement or fusion depending on the patient's age and preoperative range of motion at the affected level.

In the last two decades, numerous cervical disc prostheses have been developed (Figs. 7.1, 7.2, 7.3, 7.4, and 7.5). Main criteria for the implantation of these relatively expensive implants are a good range of motion at the affected level in preoperative functional X-ray images and a biological age of less than 55 years. Furthermore, the level of osteochondrosis in preoperative CT scans and MRIs is taken into account.

A historical overview about the development of cervical disc prostheses is given in Sect. 1.2. The most widespread model of the first generation was the Prodisc-C prosthesis (Synthes, Umkirch, Germany). Numerous spine surgeons criticised the difficult implantation procedure due to the big keels in the endplates. This fact was taken into

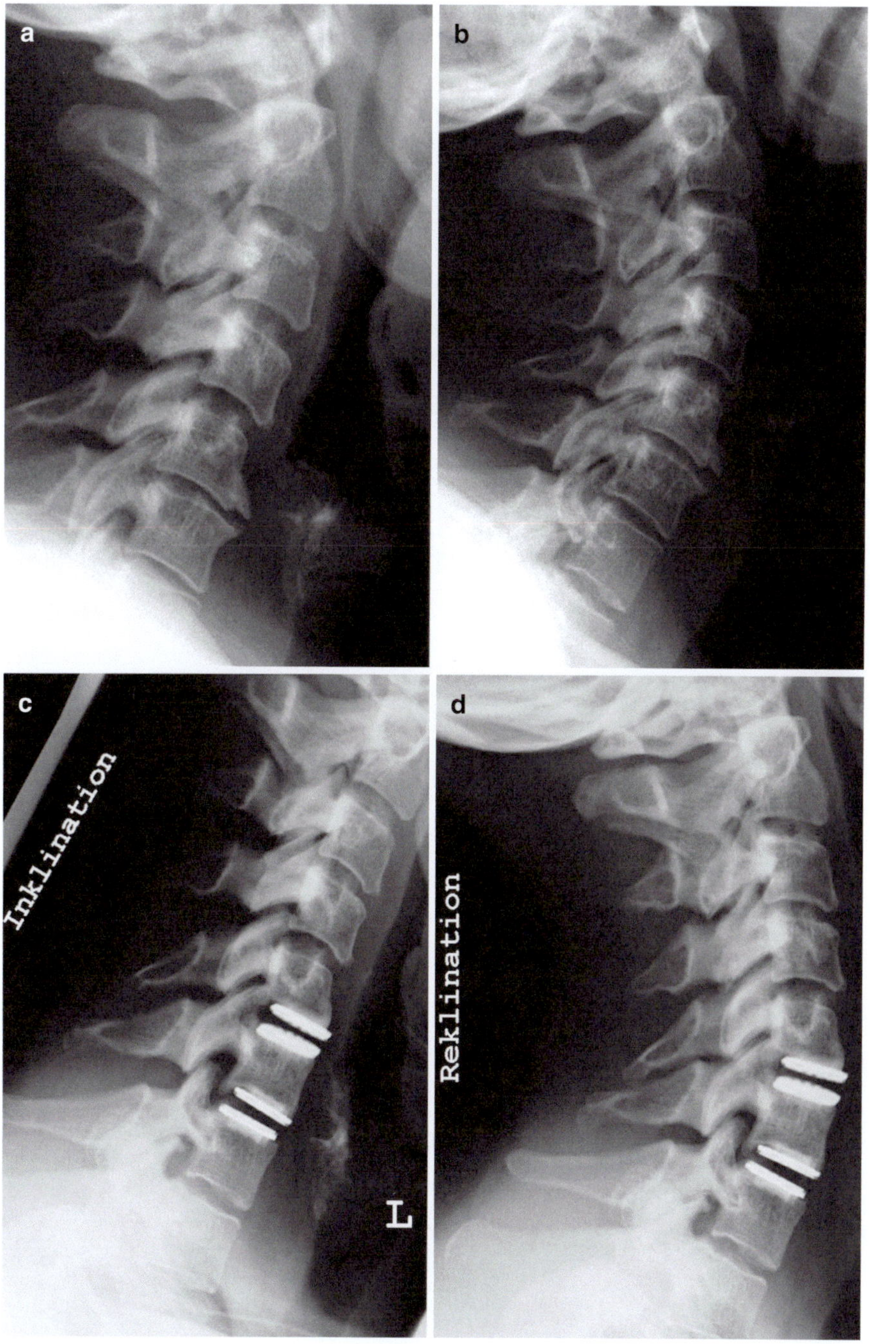

Fig. 7.3 Symptomatic osteochondrosis at C5/6 and disc herniation at C6/7 in a 45-year-old patient. Preoperative lateral functional X-ray studies in flexion (**a**) and extension (**b**) show a minimum residual range of motion at the affected levels. Intraoperatively improved motion due to resection of osteophytes, therefore total disc replacement with M6C prostheses (Spinal Kinetics, Sunnyvale, USA) at both levels. Postoperative lateral functional X-ray studies in flexion (**c**) and extension (**d**)

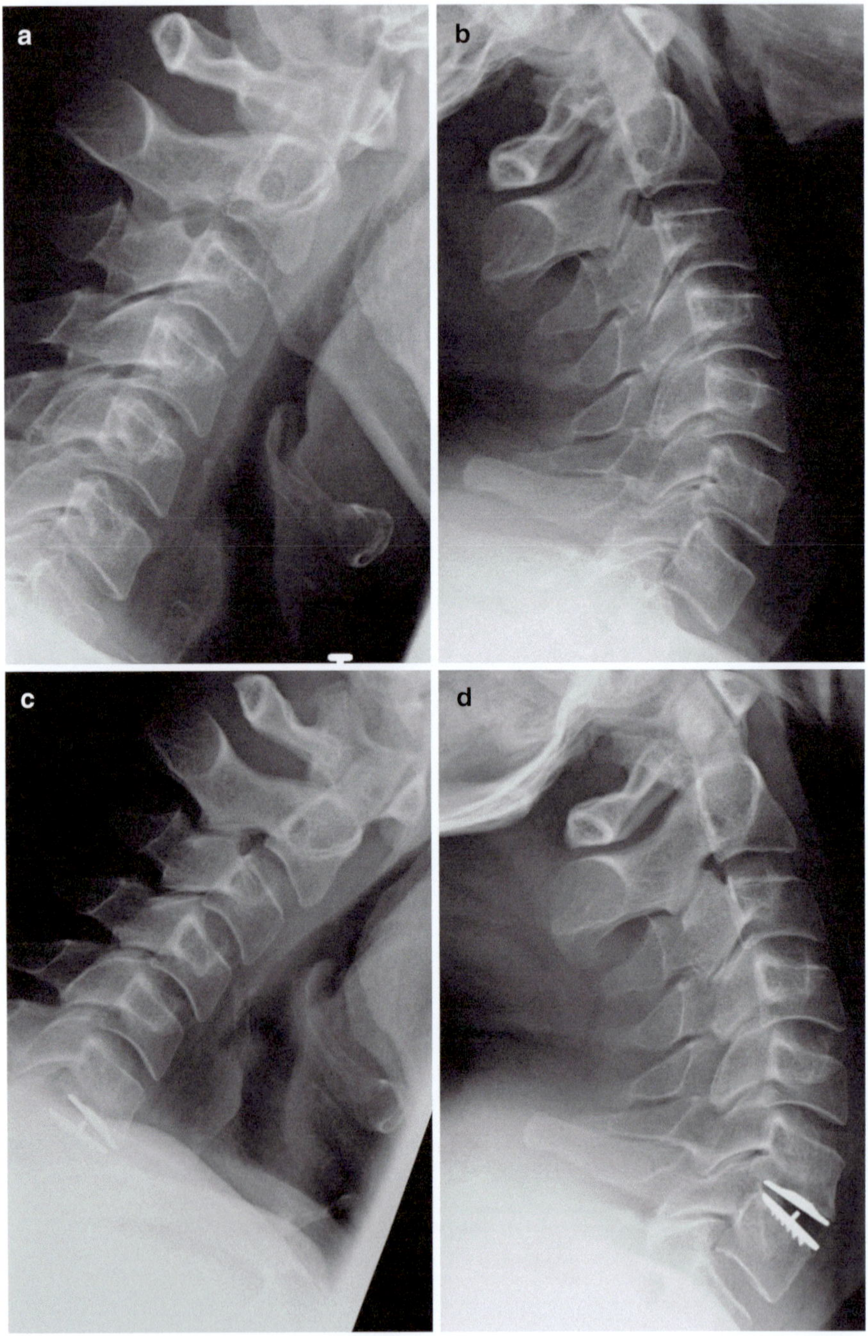

Fig. 7.4 Symptomatic disc herniation at C6/7 in a 42-year-old patient. Good range of motion at the affect level in preoperative functional lateral X-ray studies in flexion (**a**) and extension (**b**), therefore total disc replacement with a Mobi-C prosthesis (LDR Medical, Rosières Prês Troyes, France). Postoperative lateral functional X-ray studies in flexion (**c**) and extension (**d**)

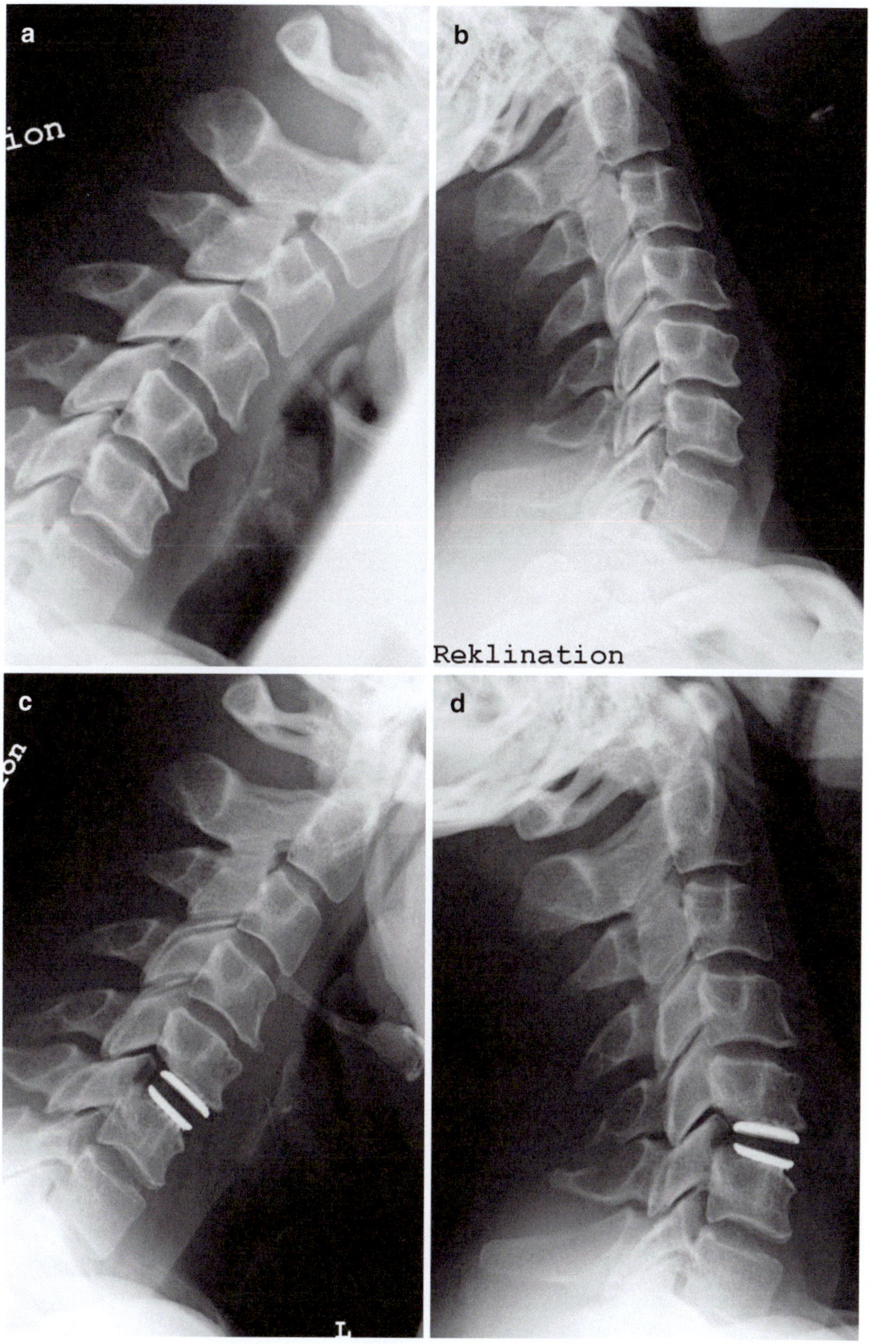

Fig. 7.5 Symptomatic disc herniation at C5/6 in a 46-year-old female patient. Good range of motion at the affected level in preoperative functional lateral X-ray studies in flexion (**a**) and extension (**b**), therefore total disc replacement with a Freedom Cervical Disc prosthesis (Axiomed, Garfield Heights, USA). Postoperative lateral functional X-ray studies in flexion (**c**) and extension (**d**)

account by the manufacturer of this implant as well as by other manufacturers (Fig. 7.1). In some cases, keels were downsized, in others, pins or teeth were added to the endplates and the prosthesis was implanted under distraction. After taking back distraction, the implant jams between the endplates of the vertebral bodies.

A widely used implant in Europe and the USA is the M6C prosthesis (Spinal Kinetics, Sunnyvale, USA; Fig. 7.2). It consists of a polyurethane core, a woven annulus made of polyethylene and endplates made of titanium, whereas the endplates have a porous surface and keels for a safe anchoring in the adjacent vertebral bodies. The handling during implantation is assessed as very good by most surgeons, and the surgical morbidity is very low. Nevertheless, the height of the prosthesis is at least 6 mm which does not always correlate with physiological conditions, especially at the anterior aspect of the vertebral bodies. The average height of the anterior intervertebral disc space is about 4 mm (see Sects. 2.1 and 2.2). Thus, it might be possible to induce overdistraction of the facet joints that can lead to persisting neck pain after surgery. Furthermore, segmental lordosis is abandoned due to the parallel titanium endplates. This fact is a disadvantage from a biomechanical point of view.

The normal anatomical shape of the intervertebral disc space with a curvature in the middle of the cranial endplate is taken into account by the latest generation of cervical disc prostheses. One example for this development was the Cadisc-C implant (Ranier, Cambridge, UK; Fig. 7.2b) with a polycarbonate polyurethane elastomere composition for the simulation of a natural disc. The biomechanical properties with six degrees of freedom and a mobile centre of rotation were similar to physiological conditions. The minimum anterior height of this implant was 4.7 mm, but it went out of production in late 2015 due to economical problems of the manufacturer. Nevertheless, it is likely that there will be more prostheses with a single-unit design in the future (Fig. 7.5).

7.1.2 Intervertebral Fusion Cages

If the patient does not meet the criteria for total disc replacement, then the implantation of an intervertebral cage is given (Fig. 7.6a and 7.7). Nowadays, many surgeons use cages made of polyetheretherketone (PEEK). The main disadvantage of this material is that it does not have osseointegrative potential. To achieve a safe fusion in the medium term, most cages have a central hole for filling it with osteoinductive substance such as tricalcium phosphate. Besides PEEK cages, numerous institutions use titanium cages that have a micro-porous surface for better osseointegration and thus a better healing. A disadvantage of these cages is the severe artefacts in postoperative MRI studies that are sometimes necessary in patients with unsatisfying clinical result of surgery. Chen et al. (2013) could show in a prospective randomised control study that PEEK cages show a better maintenance of intervertebral height and lordosis as well as clinical outcome compared to titanium cages. Nevertheless, there is a recent trend to titanium cages to avoid the filling of the cage with osteoinductive substances and because of their excellent osseointegration.

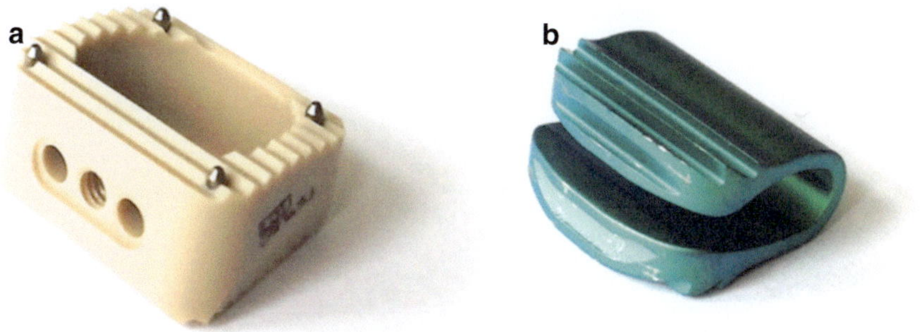

Fig. 7.6 Shell cage (Advanced Medical Technologies, Meerbusch, Germany) with a central opening for filling with osteoinductive material to achieve a bony fusion (**a**). Dynamic Cervical Implant DCI (Paradigm Spine, Wurmlingen, Germany) made of titanium allowing flexion and extension movements in the sagittal plane (**b**)

The implantation of intervertebral cages without additional anterior plating in one-level and two-level case is the most frequent method to achieve cervical fusion at most European neurosurgical departments. However most orthopaedic spine surgeons tend to use additional anterior plating on a regular base. The authors' use anterior plating after cage implantation at three or more levels only.

7.1.3 Intermediate Solution

Besides the use of cages or prostheses, there is the possibility of an intermediate solution with the so-called dynamic cervical implant DCI (Paradigm Spine, Wurmlingen, Germany) which allows motions in the sagittal plane (flexion and extension; Figs. 7.6b and 7.8).

7.1.4 Hybrid Solutions

In cases of two-level and three-level surgeries, it is possible to establish a hybrid solution with a combination of cage and prosthesis (Fig. 7.9). This method achieved very good clinical and radiological results in several studies (Barbagallo et al. 2009; König et al. 2015; Shin et al. 2009; Spetzger et al. 2013).

7.1.5 Polymethylmethacrylate (PMMA)

In the last three decades, numerous cervical fusions after discectomy have been done by using PMMA. Early experimental and clinical evaluations of PMMA interposition were published by Roosen (1982). It could be shown that despite the heat

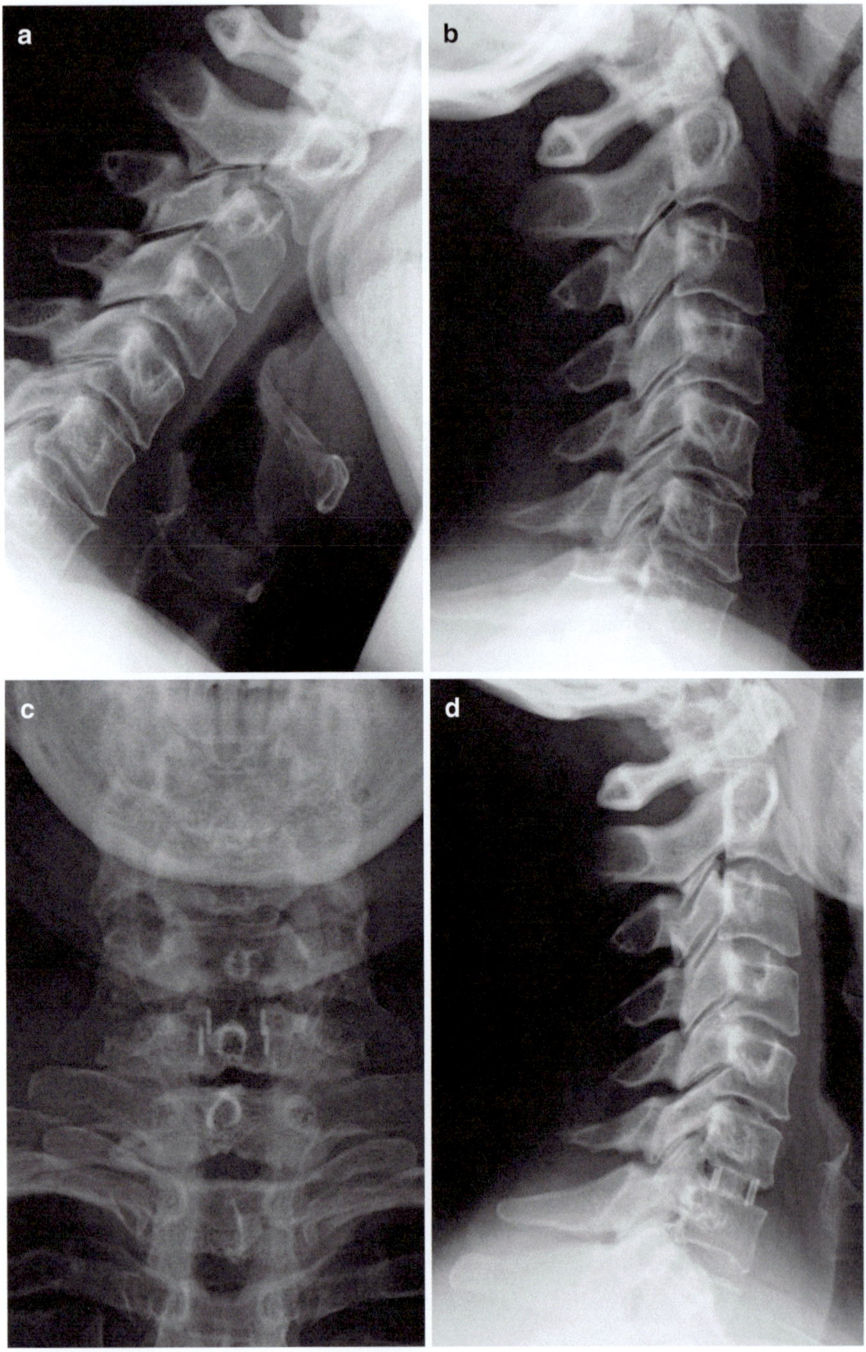

Fig. 7.7 Osteochondrosis at C6/7 with consecutive radiculopathy in a 46-year-old female patient. Lack of motion at the affected level in preoperative lateral X-ray studies in flexion (**a**) and extension (**b**), therefore implantation of a cervical fusion cage. X-ray studies after surgery, anterior-posterior (**c**) and lateral (**d**) images

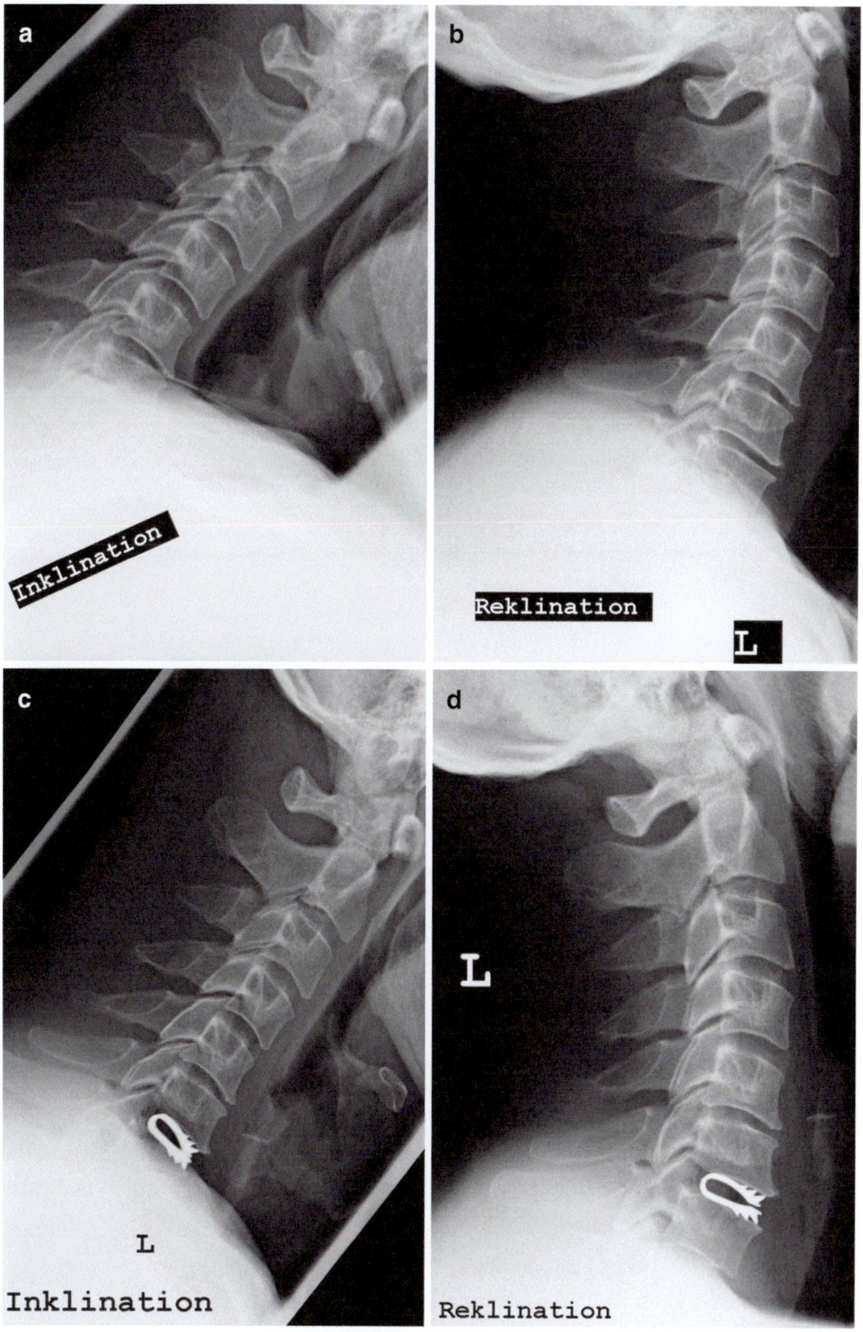

Fig. 7.8 A 45-year-old patient with a symptomatic disc herniation at C6/7. Preoperative lateral functional X-ray studies (**a**, **b**). The affected level cannot be assessed in flexion (**a**). In extension loss of height of the disc space as a sign of mild osteochondrosis (**b**). Intraoperatively sufficient range of motion of the affected level, therefore implantation of dynamic cervical implant DCI (Paradigm Spine, Wurmlingen, Germany) with height of 5 mm that enables flexion and extension in the sagittal plane. Postoperative lateral functional X-ray images in flexion (**c**) and extension (**d**)

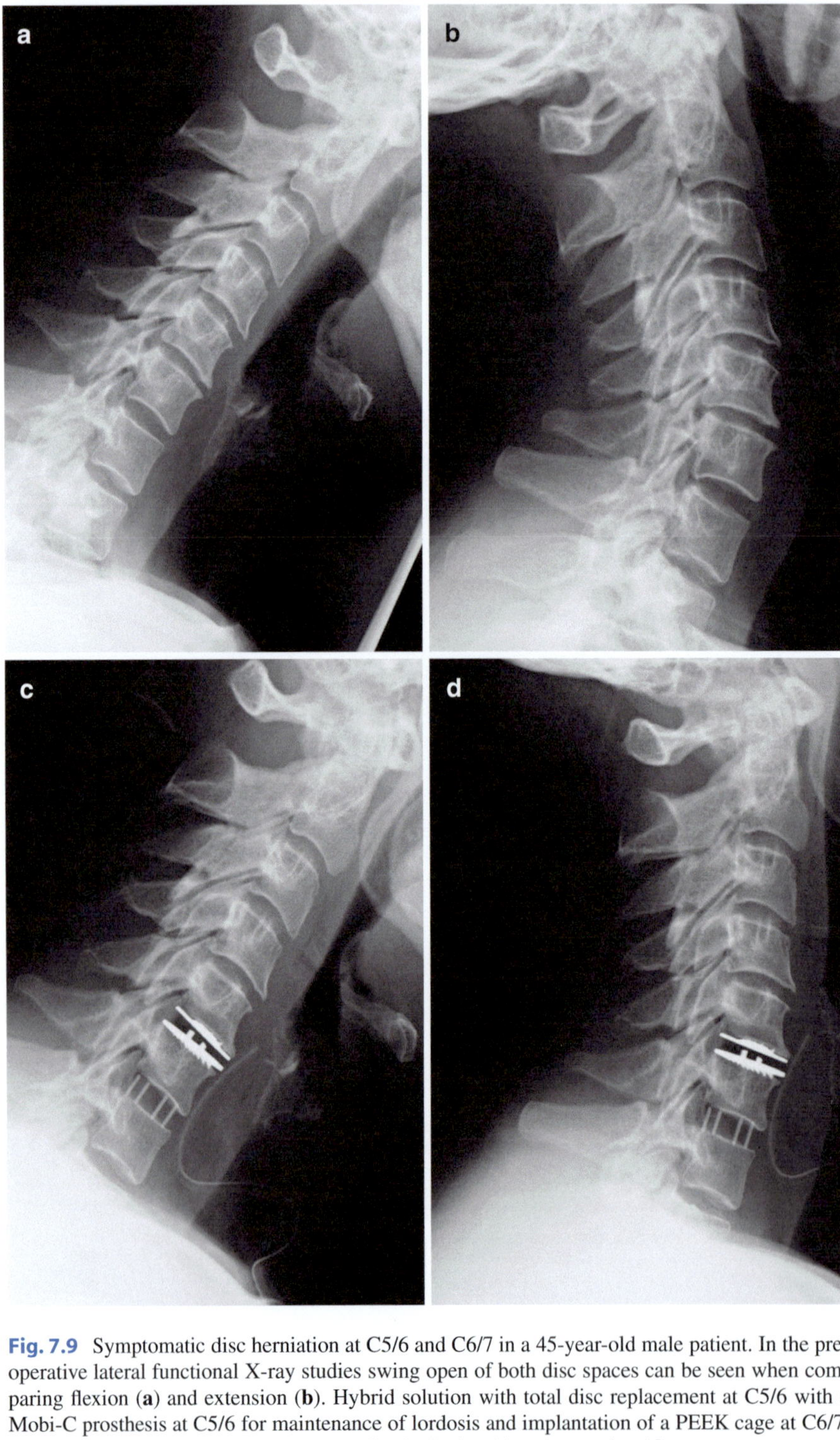

Fig. 7.9 Symptomatic disc herniation at C5/6 and C6/7 in a 45-year-old male patient. In the preoperative lateral functional X-ray studies swing open of both disc spaces can be seen when comparing flexion (**a**) and extension (**b**). Hybrid solution with total disc replacement at C5/6 with a Mobi-C prosthesis at C5/6 for maintenance of lordosis and implantation of a PEEK cage at C6/7. Postoperative lateral functional X-ray studies in flexion (**c**) and extension (**d**)

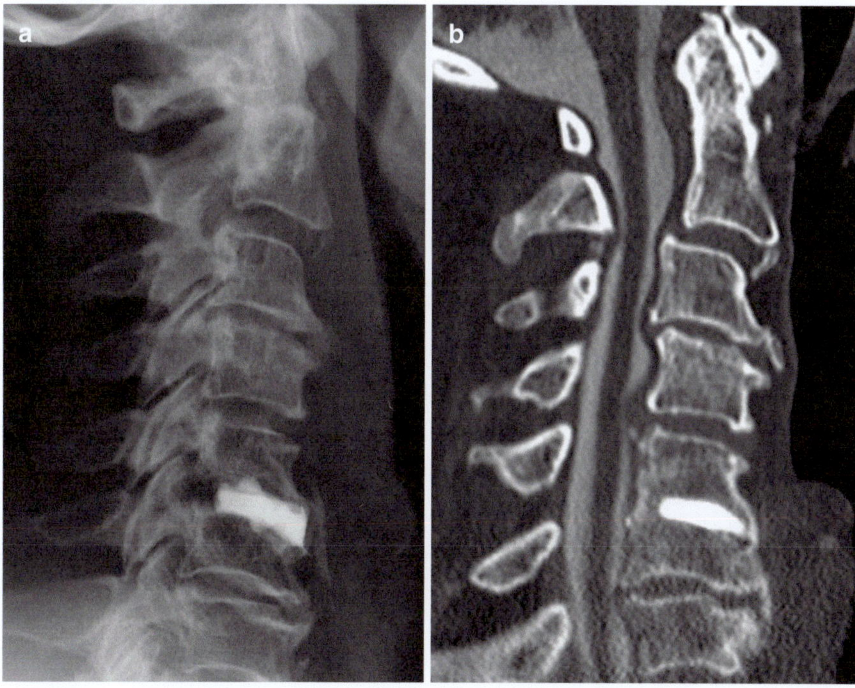

Fig. 7.10 Interposition of PMMA after discectomy at C5/6. Lateral X-ray image 1 day after surgery (**a**). Bony fusion around the PMMA 3 years after surgery in a sagittal CT scan (**b**)

generation during the hardening of the PMMA, there is no necrosis in the surrounding soft tissue including the neural tissue.

By using this technique with grouting of the intervertebral disc space, the surgeon creates an optimum, patient-individualised surface. Nowadays, PMMA is occasionally used when even the smallest cages are too high to fit in a very narrow disc space. Compared to cages and prostheses the use of PMMA is very low-priced.

In the long term after PMMA application, good clinical results with either fusion (Fig. 7.10) or persisting minimum pseudarthrosis have been observed. The supporter of PMMA use refers to the low clinical relevance of the pseudarthroses (Fig. 7.11).

7.1.6 Autologous Iliac Crest Bone Graft and Anterior Plating

The classical surgical technique with implantation of a cylindrical bone graft from the iliac crest was established by Cloward (1958). Additional anterior plating was introduced to avoid secondary subsidence of the bone graft (Caspar et al. 1989; Hermann 1975). This classical surgical technique is still used in cases of osteochondrosis and/or disc herniation without instability in the Anglo-American countries.

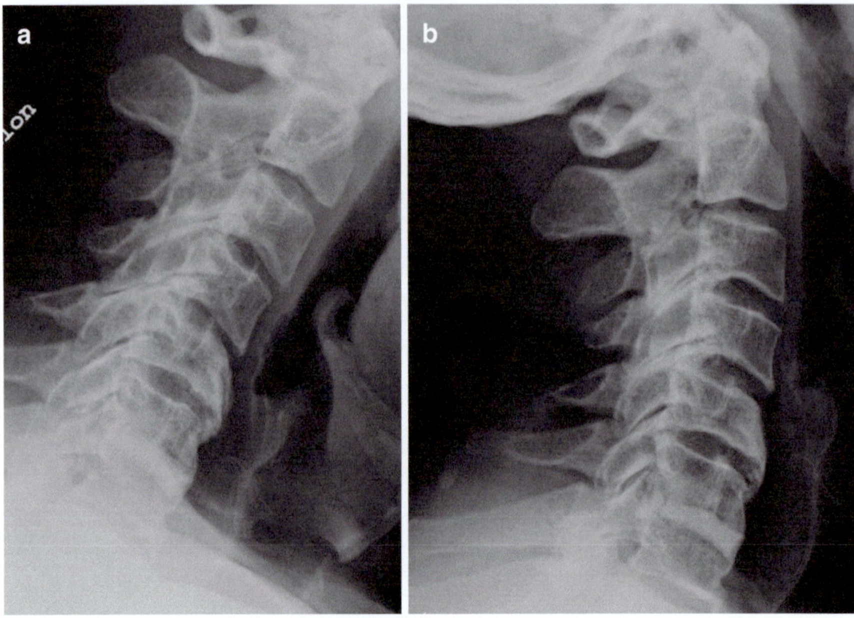

Fig. 7.11 PMMA interposition after discectomy at C6/7. Minimal motions in comparison of flexion (**a**) and extension (**b**) in lateral functional X-ray studies due to a pseudarthrosis. Since the patient completely recovered from his C7 radicular syndrome, there was no indication for revision surgery

Besides that, it is still a safe procedure in cases of degenerative instability with rupture of the intervertebral disc (Fig. 7.12). For the treatment of traumatic instability, a discectomy with interposition of an iliac crest bone graft and anterior plating is still the therapeutical gold standard.

7.1.7 Cages with Screw Fixation

Besides the numerous stand-alone cages with or without pins at the endplates that are implanted into the disc space under distraction, there is a solution with fixing of the cage by angled screws called Zero P (Synthes, Oberdorf, Switzerland; Fig. 7.13). In the authors' opinion, its implantation is indicated if there is degenerative instability next to a previous anterior fusion in adjacent levels (Fig. 7.13b). In this case, the use of this fixable cage is of advantage because the previous anterior plate can be left in place which avoids surgical morbidity due to removal of the plate.

7.1.8 Clinical Case: Indication for Total Disc Replacement

A 49-year-old patient was admitted to our department with a history of neck pain and brachialgia for 3 months. These clinical complaints were progressive despite

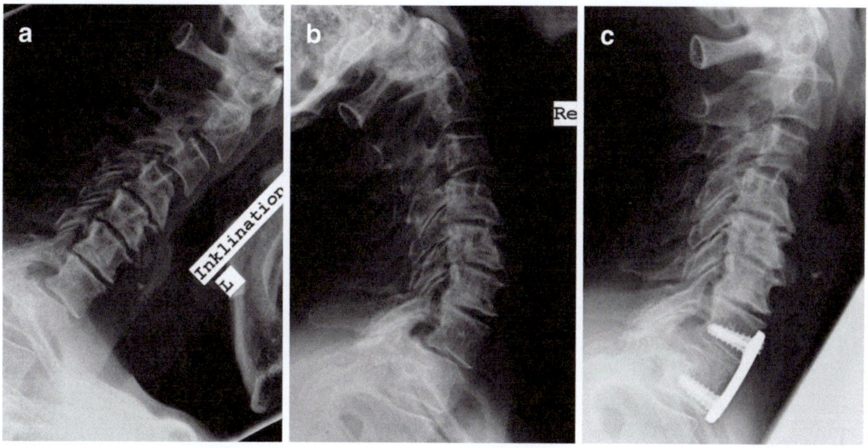

Fig. 7.12 Degenerative spinal instability at C7/T1 in lateral functional X-ray studies in flexion (**a**) and extension (**b**). Postoperative lateral X-ray image after fusion with a iliac crest bone graft and anterior plating (**c**)

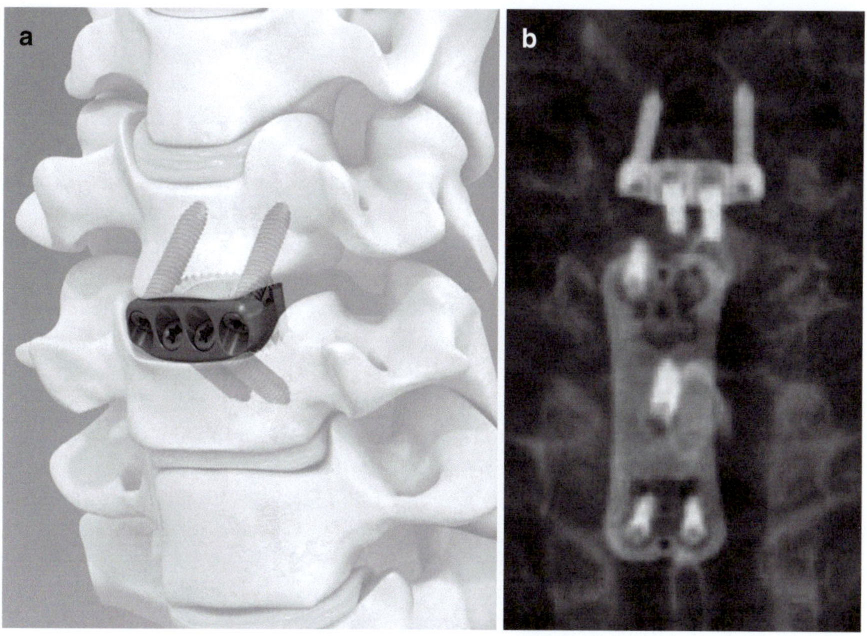

Fig. 7.13 Zero P cage with screw fixation (**a**; with kind permission by Synthes, Umkirch, Germany). Implantation of this cage is indicated for fusion surgery adjacent to a previous fusion with an anterior plate, anterior-posterior X-ray image (**b**)

conservative treatment. The past medical history included fusion at C6/7 with PMMA 10 years ago. In the clinical examination, paresthesia in the right C6 dermatome and a slight palsy of the right biceps muscle (grade 4 of 5) were verified. The biceps reflex was weak on the right side and normal on the left side. Coordination tests (Unterberger's stepping test, tightrope walking test) were normal. The sensation of vibration as well as the reflexes of the lower limbs showed physiological findings as well. There were no signs of disorders of the pyramidal tracts; thus, we could not find clinical signs of spinal cord compression.

MRI of the cervical spine showed slight osteochondrosis and a right-sided disc herniation with consecutive compression of the right C6 nerve root at the level of C5/6 (Fig. 7.14). Preoperative lateral functional X-ray images showed a good range of motion at the affected level. After failure of conservative treatment, the indication for total disc replacement with the aim of maintenance of motion and segmental lordosis was established.

The intraoperative measurement of the intervertebral disc space brought the indication for implantation of a cervical prosthesis with the following dimensions:

- Anterior height: 4.8 mm
- Central height: 6.5 mm
- Posterior height: 3.6 mm
- Widest lateral width: 17 mm
- Anterior-posterior depth: 13.3 mm

Postoperative lateral functional X-ray images showed an adequate position of the cervical prosthesis. The patient reported about remission of neck pain and brachialga already at the first day after surgery, the weakness of the right biceps muscle was still detectable (grade 4+ of 5). Physiotherapy in an outpatient facility was prescribed to support the good postoperative clinical result.

7.1.9 Clinical Case: Indication for Cage Implantation

A 52-year-old female patient was admitted to our institution with head and neck pain and a right-sided brachialgia (mainly radiating to the shoulder) for the last 4 months. Clinical complaints persisted despite conservative treatment.

The clinical examination showed paresthesia in the right C5 dermatome and a weakness of the right deltoid muscle (grade 4 of 5). The brachioradialis reflex was weak on the right side and normal on the left side. Coordination tests (Unterberger's stepping test, tightrope walking test) did not show any ataxia. The sensation of vibration as well as the reflexes of the lower limbs showed physiological findings as well. There were no signs of disorders of the pyramidal tracts; thus, we could not find clinical signs of spinal cord compression.

MRI of the cervical spine showed mild osteochondrosis at C4/5 with consecutive narrowing of the spinal canal and the neuroforamina (predominant on the right side; Fig. 7.15). Preoperative lateral functional X-ray studies did not show significant residual motion at the affected level C4/5 but a synostosis at C2/3. Due to the failure of conservative treatment, we saw an indication for discectomy, decompression of neural structures and implantation of a cervical fusion cage. The cage was filled

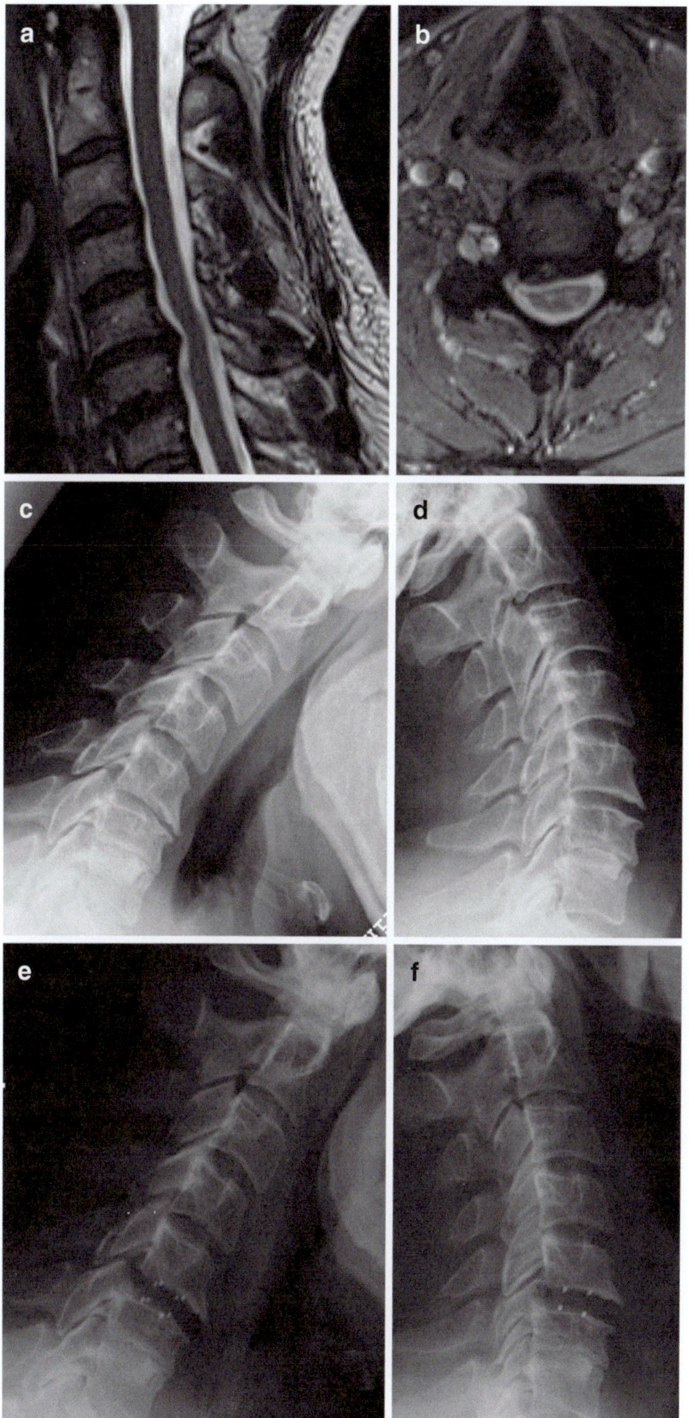

Fig. 7.14 Osteochondrosis and disc herniation at C5/6 after PMMA fusion at C6/7 10 years earlier. MRI in sagittal (**a**) and axial (**b**) plane. Preoperative lateral functional X-ray studies in flexion (**c**) and extension (**d**). Postoperative lateral functional X-ray studies in flexion (**e**) and extension (**f**) after total disc replacement at C5/6 with a Cadisc-C prosthesis

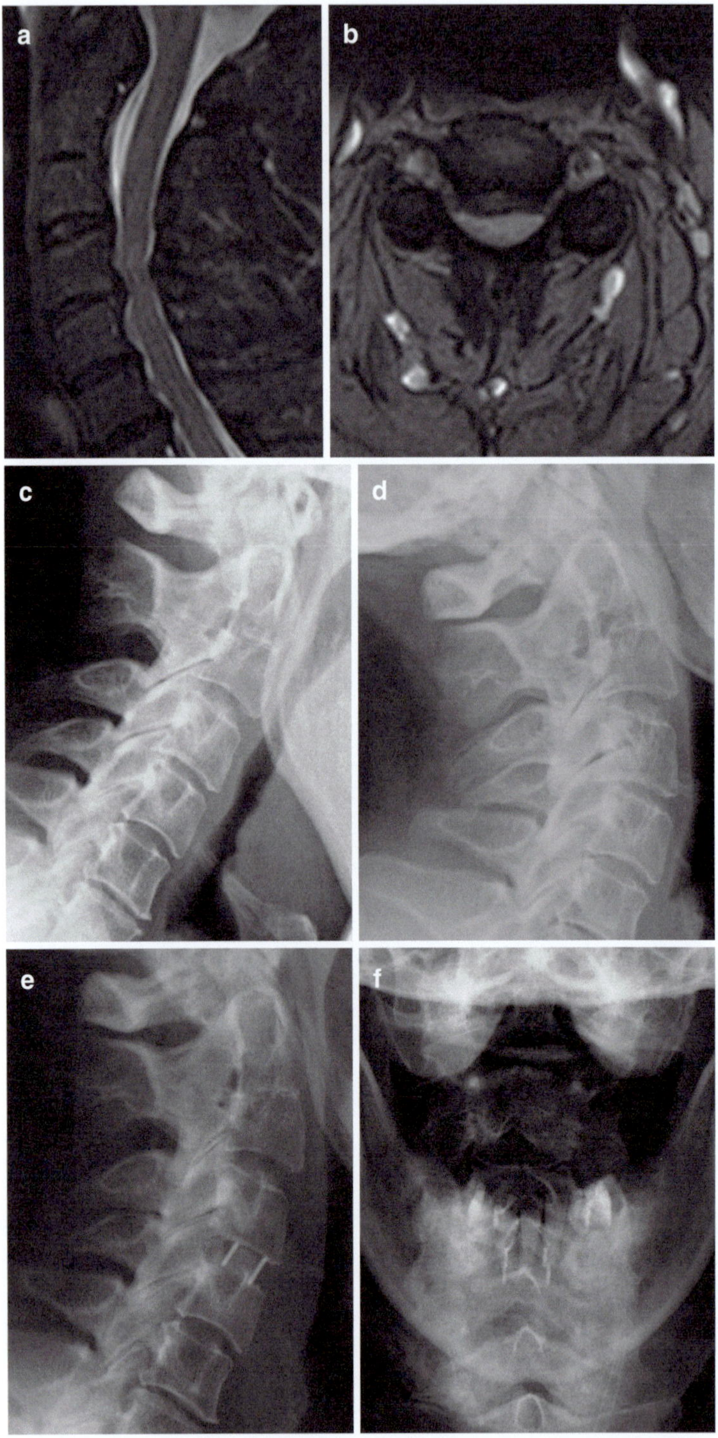

Fig. 7.15 Broad-based osteochondrosis at C4/5 and synostosis at C2/3, MRI in sagittal (**a**) and axial (**b**) planes. Preoperative lateral functional X-ray studies in flexion (**c**) and extension (**d**) without significant motion at C4/5. Postoperative lateral functional X-ray studies in flexion (**e**) and extension (**f**) after implantation of a PEEK cage to achieve secondary bony fusion

the with osteoinductive material Vitoss (Stryker, Dosburg, Germany) to achieve bony fusion of the adjacent vertebral bodies. Postoperative X-ray studies in two planes showed a good reestablishment of the intervertebral height in the degenerated level and a correct position of the cage Compact Cornerstone (Medtronic, Meerbusch, Germany).

The patient reported about subtotal regression of head and neck pain as well as brachialgia already at the first day after surgery. The weakness of the right deltoid muscle showed partial recovery (grade 4+ of 5). Physiotherapy in an outpatient facility was prescribed to support the good postoperative clinical result.

7.2 Replacement of Vertebral Bodies and Anterior Plating

7.2.1 Vertebral Body Replacement

The use of an autologous iliac crest bone graft is still the gold standard for cervical vertebral body replacement (Figs. 7.18 and 8.37). By analogy to the development of cages for implantation after discectomy, the industry developed vertebral body replacements for the use after cervical corpectomy made of PEEK or titanium (Figs. 7.16, 7.17, 7.19, and 7.20). The advantage of these implants is the exclusion of surgical morbidity that is associated with bone harvesting at the iliac crest: haematoma, infection, fracture or nerve lesion (Epstein 2012; König and Spetzger 2014). The fusion rate of these implants is according to several studies approximately close to that of autologous bone (Epstein 2012; Medow et al. 2006). Nevertheless, most publications refer to titanium implants. The main disadvantage of both alloplastic materials are the relatively high costs. Furthermore, there are reports about a higher rate of subsidence of PEEK cages into adjacent vertebral bodies in the long term which correlates with the authors' experience (König et al. 2013).

Distractable or adjustable titanium cages like the ADD and ADD plus implants (Ulrich medical, Ulm, Germany) can be easily adjusted in situ to the required height. Due to the optional fixation of the ADD plus model, the surgical procedure is simplified since an additional anterior plating is unnecessary (Fig. 7.16). The Ulrich implants can be used for defects up to 65 mm. This is usually sufficient for the replacement of three cervical vertebral bodies; however, an additional posterior fusion is recommended because of the high biomechanical stresses in these cases (Kim and Alexander 2006). A possible disadvantage of multilevel vertebral body replacement with the ADD or ADD plus implants is the lack of the physiological lordosis.

The PEEK implant ATHLET (Signus, Alzenau, Germany) can be adjusted to a height up to 50 mm by combining two PEEK elements after measuring the corpectomy defect. A central opening enables the possibility of filling the implant with autologous bone from the corpectomy or the osteoinductive bioceramic material KAINOS (Signus, Alzenau, Germany).

The choice of the adequate vertebral body replacement basically depends on the surgeon's preferences. At the authors' institution, the iliac crest bone graft is

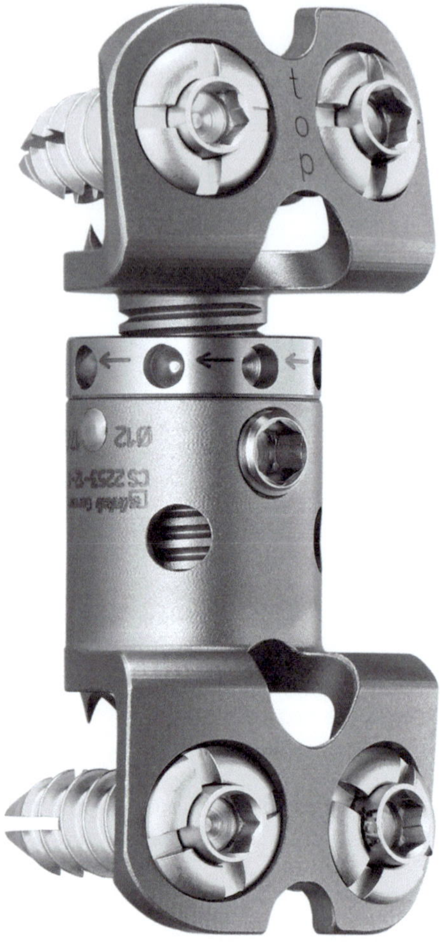

Fig. 7.16 Distractable titanium vertebral body replacement ADDplus (with kind permission by ulrich medical, Ulm, Germany)

preferred because of its excellent fusion rate and its low costs (Fig. 7.18). For revision surgeries or cases where bone harvesting has to be avoided for medical reasons (osteoporosis, renal failure, underlying malign disease), we prefer distractable titanium cages.

7.2.2 Anterior Plating

Nowadays, there are numerous systems for anterior plating of the cervical spine on the market. Titanium is the standard material for osteosynthesis since it combines optimum properties like high fixedness, resistance to corrosion and extreme temperatures as well as low mass. There are no reports about immunological rejection. Osseointegration of titanium is very high (Assad et al. 2003a, b; Borsari et al. 2007; Slivka et al. 2006).

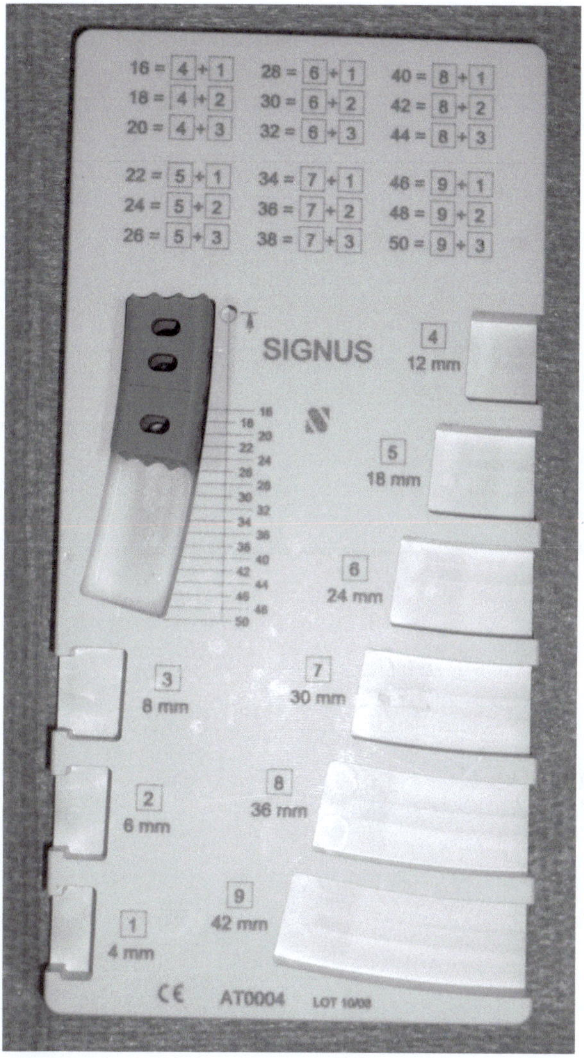

Fig. 7.17 Vertebral body replacement ATHLET™ made of PEEK. The height of the implant can be adjusted in 2-mm steps by combining two PEEK bodies

The surgical procedure of anterior plating is simplified by self-drilling screws making pre-drilling and thread cutting unnecessary. Thus, with less operating steps the X-ray dose per operation decreases.

The highest stability of an anterior plating construct is achieved by bicortical screws. Expanding screws did not achieve recognition in cervical spinal surgery since a higher rate of subsidence and dislocation, especially in combination with a PEEK vertebral body replacement, had been observed (König and Spetzger 2014).

Typical dimensions of screws for cervical anterior plating are as follows:

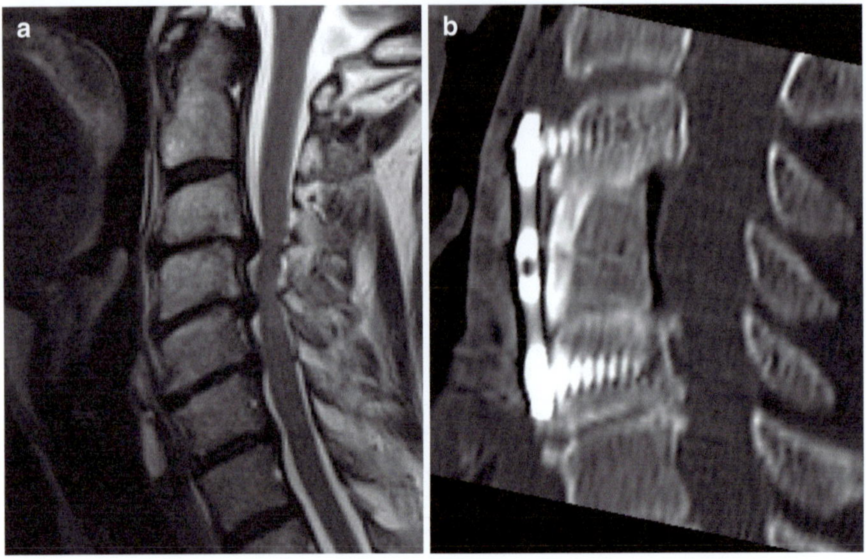

Fig. 7.18 Spinal stenosis at C3/4 and C4/5 with space-occupying degenerative changes at the anterior aspect of the spinal cord, sagittal MRI (**a**). Indication for corpectomy, decompression, implantation of an iliac crest bone graft, and anterior plating with the Skyline™ system, sagittal CT scan (**b**)

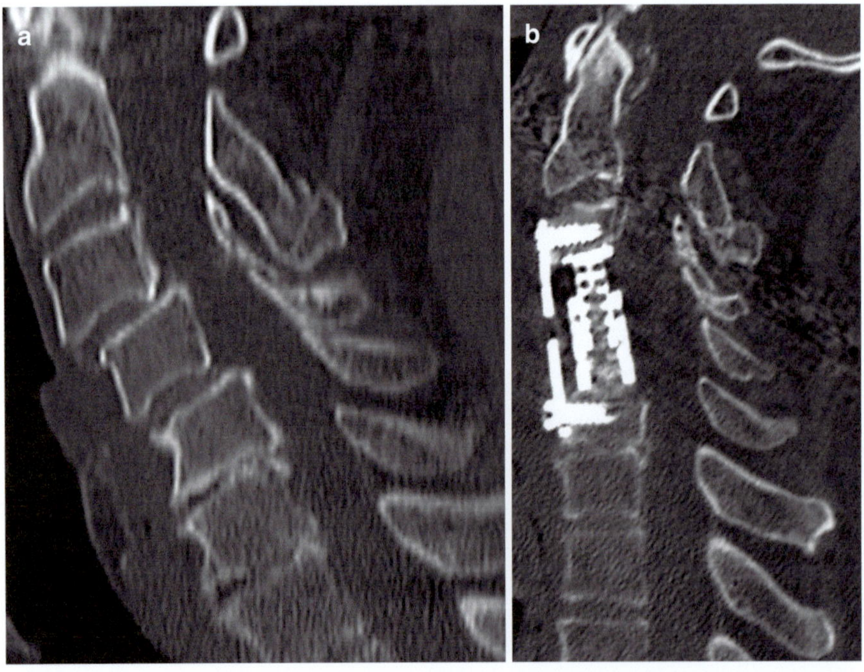

Fig. 7.19 Degenerative spinal instability with consecutive spinal stenosis from the C3 to the C5 vertebral body in a 73-year-old male patient, sagittal CT scan (**a**). Indication for corpectomy of C4, decompression, vertebral body replacement with the ADDplus™ implant, and anterior plating; sagittal CT scan (**b**)

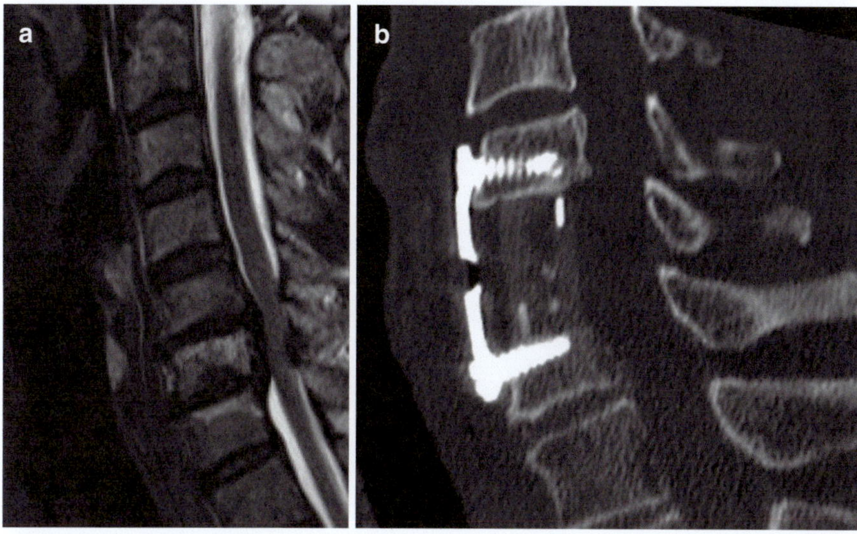

Fig. 7.20 Osteoligamentous spinal stenosis from the C5 to the C7 vertebral body in a 56-year-old male patient, sagittal MRI (**a**). Indication for corpectomy of C6, decompression, vertebral body replacement with the ATHLET™ implant, and anterior plating; sagittal CT scan (**b**). The implant had been filled with autologous bone chips and osteoinductive bioceramic KAINOS™ (Signus, Alzenau, Germany)

- A diameter of 4.0 mm for standard screws and 4.5 mm for revision screws
- A length of 14–18 mm for monocortical screws (dependent on the anterior-posterior dimensions of the vertebral body and the placement angle in the sagittal and axial planes)
- A length of 18–22 mm for bicortical screws (also dependent on the anterior-posterior dimensions of the vertebral body and the placement angle in the sagittal and axial planes)

The industry offers fixed angle as well as variable angle locking plate systems, whereas there are no clear recommendations for the several indications. In clinical practice, usually fixed angle locking plates are used for traumatic instabilities since structures of the posterior column (vertebral arches, facet joints, roots of vertebral arches) are often fractured, too, and these plates provide maximum stability for anterior procedures.

In cases of degenerative instabilities, most surgeons use variable angle plate systems (Hong et al. 2010). In these cases, segmental instability is much less compared to traumatic instabilities because posterior load-bearing structures are usually intact. Furthermore, the lateral walls of the vertebral bodies can be usually left in place during corpectomy for decompression of the spinal canal, and thus the amount of instability is relatively low. The angle variable locking plates allow micro-movements that are supposed to be of advantage for the fusion of iliac crest bone graft and vertebral bodies of the adjacent vertebrae.

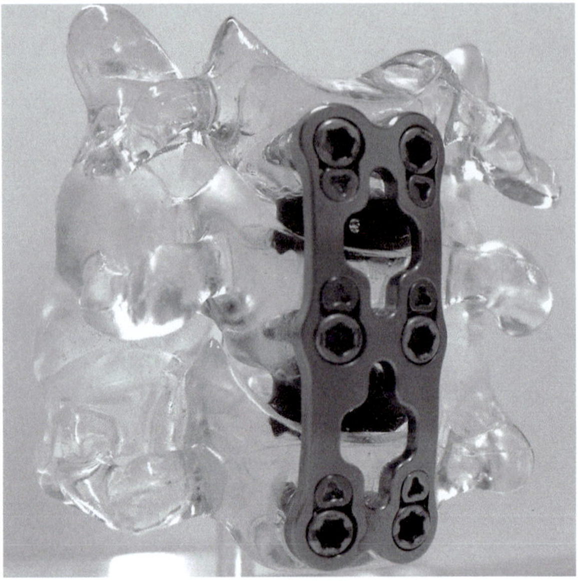

Fig. 7.21 Anterior plating system Skyline™ with locking mechanism (smaller screws) for fixing of the screw heads (With kind permission by Synthes, Umkirch, Germany)

For a higher safety of surgery, there are guiding instruments that provide an optimum angle for screw insertion in the axial plane, for example in the Skyline system (DePuy GmbH, Kirkel, Germany) that provides a free angle in the sagittal plane and a convergence of degrees in the axial plane.

In the same system, screws can be fixed with a special locking mechanism to avoid migration of a screw or loosening of the plate (Fig. 7.21). Furthermore, if revision surgery is necessary the locking mechanism can be opened again and the plate relatively easy be removed.

Due to the continuous development of plating systems, the implants have a very flat profile that avoids swallowing disorders after anterior plating surgery (Fig. 7.22).

7.2.3 Clinical Case: Indication for Vertebral Body Replacement and Anterior Plating

A 68-year-old female patient was admitted to the emergency department of our hospital because she had been unable to walk for 2 days. Before that, walking was only possible with aid. She reported about a temporary sensation of needles and pins on both arms as well as hypaesthesia of the distal right leg. In the clinical examination, a high-grade tetraparesis with dominance on the right side was found. There was a hyperreflexia of all reflexes on both legs. Nevertheless, Babinski's sign was negative on both sides. Furthermore, there were no vegetative disorders.

Emergency MRI of the spinal column showed a massive anterior compression of the spinal cord from C5 to C7 due to osteochondrosis with disc herniations (Fig. 7.23a). Because of the tetraparesis, we saw an emergency indication for decompression of

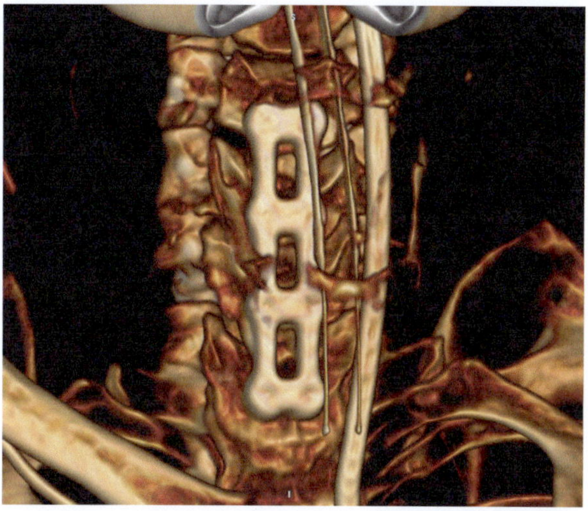

Fig. 7.22 3D reconstruction of a postoperative CT scan showing anterior plating from the C3 to the C6 vertebra after corpectomy of C4 and C5

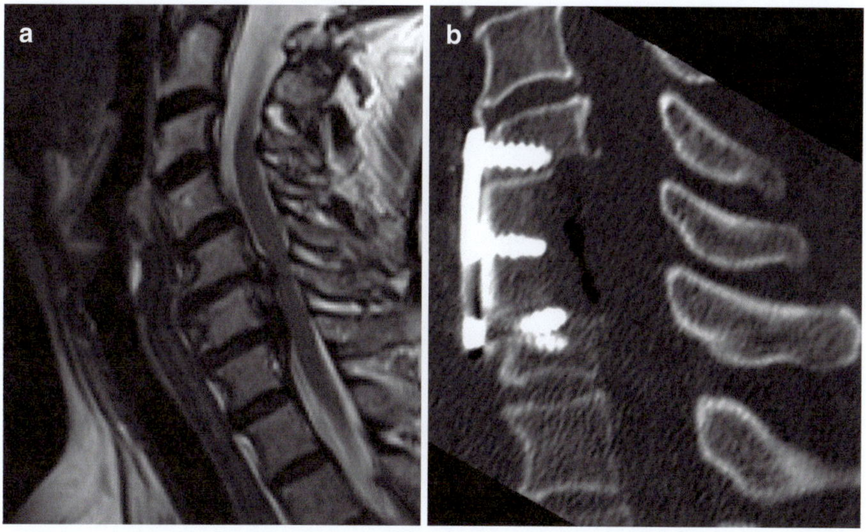

Fig. 7.23 Confluent spinal stenosis with compression of the spinal cord from C5 to C7 in a 68-year-old female patient, sagittal MRI (**a**). Indication for corpectomy of C6, decompression, implantation of an iliac crest bone graft, and anterior plating from C5 to C7; sagittal CT scan (**b**)

the spinal cord by corpectomy of the C6 vertebra with vertebral body replacement and anterior plating. Surgery was performed at the day of admission.

A postoperative CT scan showed a correct position of the implants (Fig. 7.23b). Thus, the patient could be re-mobilised under physiotherapeutical treatment. Already after a week, she was able to walk without aid. There was only a slight ataxia of the lower limbs. The upper limbs did not have any palsies, and coordination was normal. Two weeks after surgery, the patient was admitted to a neurological rehab clinic.

7.3 Posterior Fusion

7.3.1 Implants

The continuous development of cervical posterior fusion systems has lead to very user-friendly systems (Komotar 2006) with self-cutting polyaxial screws, reposition instruments, variable transverse connectors, etc., for example, the Synapse™ system by Synthes (Umkirch, Germany).

Posterior fusion systems consist of titanium alloy (including 6 % of aluminium and 7 % of niobium) because of the positive biocompatible properties of this material (compare Sect. 7.2).

The dimensions of lateral mass screws are often a diameter of 3.5 mm and a length of 10–16 mm. The proper length of the screws depends on the individual anatomical conditions, the size of the lateral mass and thus the level and size of the vertebra. Therefore, the lateral mass of C6 is much bigger than that of C3. For C7 and the upper thoracic vertebrae, pedicle screws are used because of the angle for lateral mass screws at C7 is unfavourable and because of the different anatomical shape of thoracic vertebrae compared to cervical vertebrae. The length of pedicle screws in the cervicothoracic area usually varies between 20 and 30 mm.

For posterior fusion systems, a top loading design was established. This means that the further construct is build up in the heads of the polyaxial screws. At first, the connecting rods are placed in the screw heads. Afterwards, they are fixed with locking screws. If a transverse connector is necessary, there is either a rod-to-rod connector or a top-loading connector (requiring higher locking screws) in the Synapse™ system (Figs. 7.24 and 7.25).

The choice of a certain system is not just influenced by the handling which has only little differences in most cases but also by the costs of the implants.

7.3.2 Clinical Case: Indication for Laminectomy and Posterior Fusion

A 58-year-old male patient was admitted to the emergency department of our hospital because he had been unable to walk for 2 days. He reported about a sensation of intense numbness in both legs.

The clinical examination showed an incomplete tetraparesis with plegia in the right leg. The left leg could be flexed in the hip joint just a little bit against gravity. Movement of the fingers was not possible on both sides. Both arms could be lifted against gravity only a little bit. The muscle tone in the upper and lower limbs was

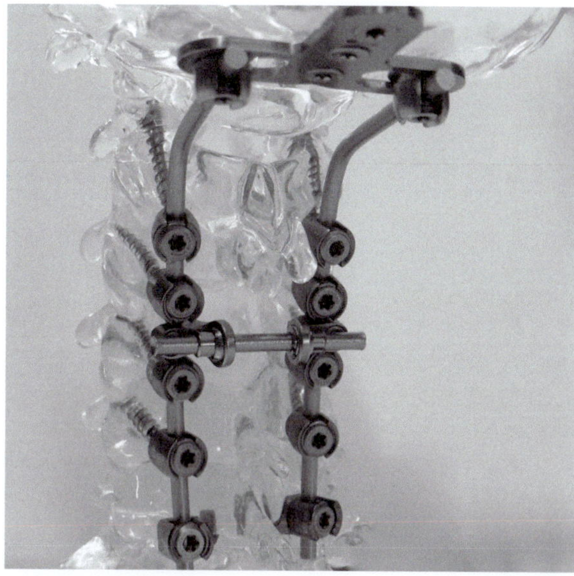

Fig. 7.24 Posterior fusion system Synapse™ with the option for occipito-cervical fusion (With kind permission of Synthes, Umkirch, Germany)

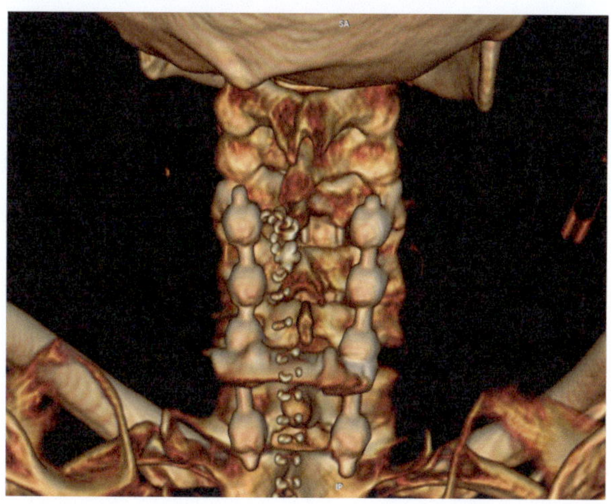

Fig. 7.25 3D reconstruction of a postoperative CT scan showing a posterior fusion from C4 to C7 with a transverse connector at the level of C6

increased with weak reflexes of the arms and hyperreflexia of the legs. Babinski's sign was positive on both sides. Hypaesthesia of both lower limbs was stated below the L1 dermatome. The patient reported about urinary incontinence.

MRI of the cervical spine showed a massive spinal stenosis from C3 to C6 due to significant degenerative changes with an extensive myelopathy signal resulting from anterior and posterior compression of the spinal cord (Fig. 7.26). The CT scan of the cervical spine showed a partial spontaneous fusion of the anterior aspects of the C3 and C4 vertebrae and a significant loss of height of the disc spaces at C3/4 and C4/5. Therefore, we saw an indication for decompression of the spinal cord by performing a laminectomy and posterior fusion particularly because the patient still

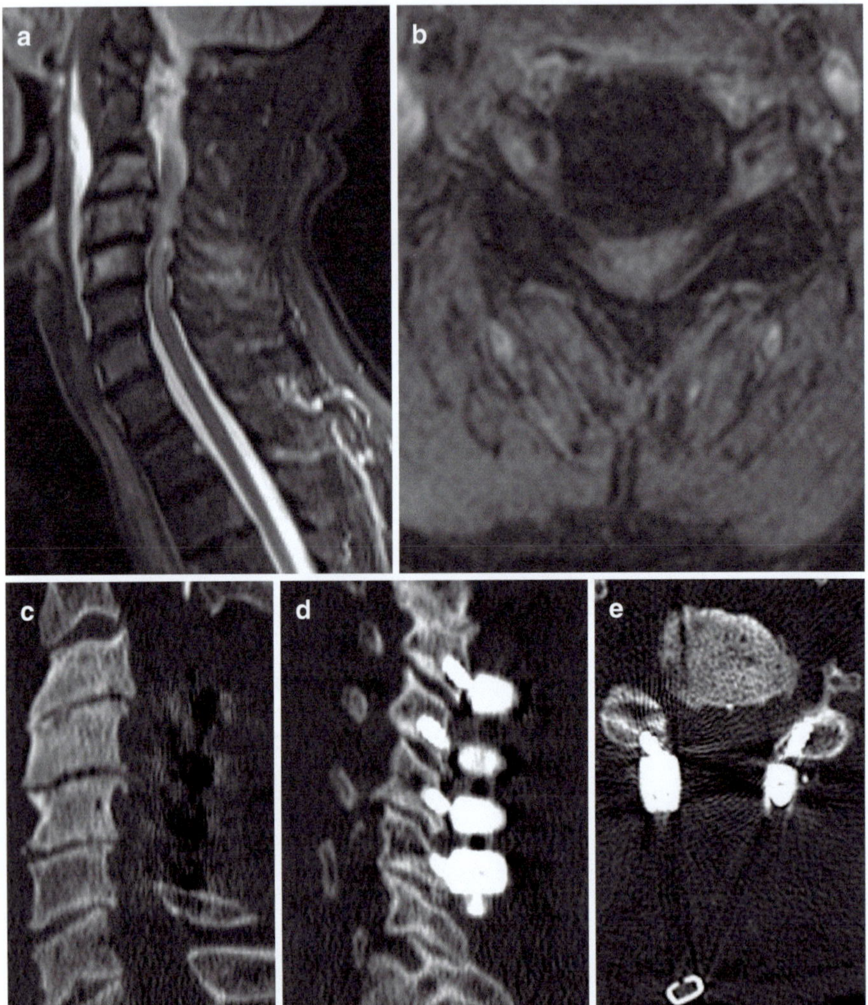

Fig. 7.26 Multilevel spinal stenosis from C3/4 to C5/6 with myelopathy signal, sagittal T2-weighted MRI (**a**). Axial MRI showing anterior compression of the spinal cord by osteochondrosis and posterior compression by hypertrophic ligaments (**b**). Indication for laminectomy and posterior fusion because of the partial bony fusion of the C3 and C4 vertebra and the narrow disc spaces at C3/4 and C4/5. Postoperative sagittal CT scan showing a good decompression of the spinal canal after laminectomy (**c**). Correct position of the lateral mass screws in a postoperative CT scan, sagittal (**d**) and axial (**e**) planes

had a good lordosis (see also Sect. 6.2). Because of the acute and severe tetraparesis, it was an emergency indication for surgery.

After surgery, the correct position of all implants could be documented by a CT scan (Fig. 7.26). The patient was slowly re-mobilised under physiotherapeutical treatment. The severe tetraparesis showed partial remission during the hospital stay, and the patient was able to walk a few steps with a Zimmer frame. The patient was referred to a rehab clinic with special emphasis on the treatment of paraplegic patients.

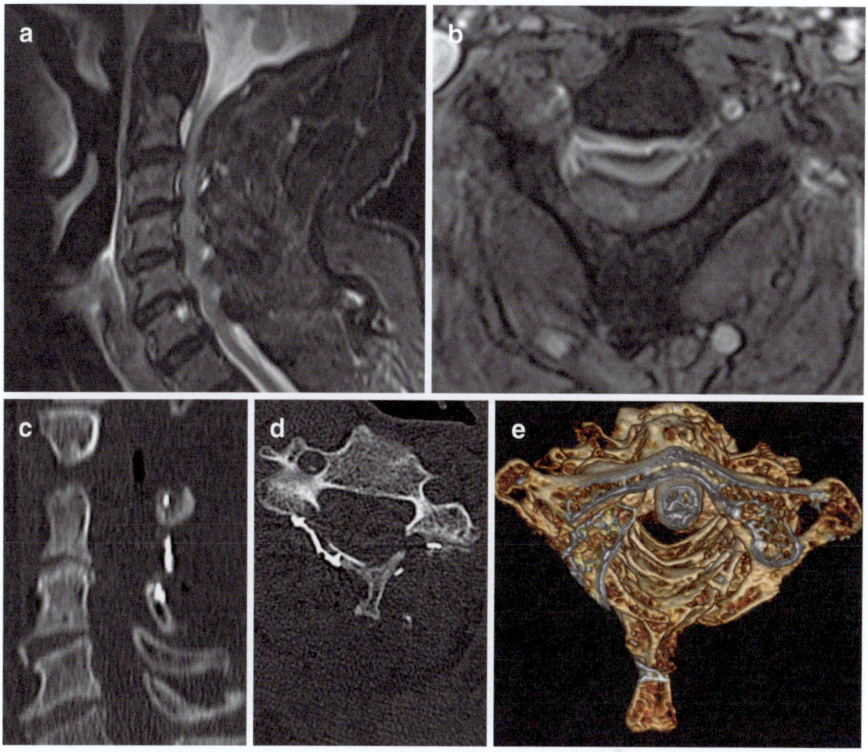

Fig. 7.27 Multilevel spinal stenosis from C2/3 to C6/7 with spinal cord compression due to dorsal ligamentous hypertrophy, MRI in the sagittal (**a**) and axial (**b**) planes. Postoperative CT scan with significant widening of the spinal canal, sagittal (**c**) and axial (**d**) planes. 3D reconstruction of the CT scan, view from cranial into the spinal canal (**e**)

7.4 Open-Door Laminoplasty

7.4.1 Implants

Besides specific fixation systems (e.g. Newbridge™ by Orthofix, Ottobrunn, Germany) that are usually quite expensive, many neurosurgeons often use miniplate fixation systems from cranial surgery, for example, the 1.5 Neuro™ titanium plate system (Biomet, Berlin, Germany).

7.4.2 Clinical Case: Indication for Open-Door Laminoplasty

A 71-year-old male patient was admitted to our outpatient clinic because he had been suffering from gait ataxia for 6 months. In the clinical examination, he presented disorders of fine motor function and sensory deficits of both hands as well as insecurity in the coordination and balance tests. The lower limbs showed hyperreflexia on both sides. Babinski's sign was negative. The patient reported that neck pain was only of slight intensity.

MRI of the cervical spine showed a massive compression of the spinal cord due to dorsal ligamentous hypertrophy (Fig. 7.27). Since functional lateral X-ray studies showed good movement despite the degeneration of the cervical spine, we indicated an open-door laminoplasty from C3 to C6 including decompression of levels C2/3 and C6/7 by using an undercutting technique.

A postoperative CT scan demonstrated an adequate decompression of the spinal canal as well as a correct position of all implants (Fig. 7.27). After surgery, the patient was re-mobilised under physiotherapeutical treatment. During the 10-day hospital stay, we did not observe any additional neurological deficits, and the patient was able to walk independently with a Zimmer frame. For further treatment, we indicated neurological rehabilitation.

References

Assad M, Chernyshov AV, Jarzem P, et al. Porous titanium-nickel for intervertebral fusion in a sheep model: part 2. Surface analysis and nickel release assessment. J Biomed Mater Res B Appl Biomater. 2003a;64(2):121–9.

Assad M, Jarzem P, Leroux MA, et al. Porous titanium-nickel for intervertebral fusion in a sheep model: part 1. Histomorphometric and radiological analysis. J Biomed Mater Res B Appl Biomater. 2003b;64(2):107–20.

Barbagallo GM, Assietti R, Corbino L, et al. Early results and review of the literature of a novel hybrid surgical technique combining cervical arthrodesis and disc arthroplasty for treating multilevel degenerative disc disease: opposite or complementary techniques? Eur Spine J. 2009;18(Suppl 1):29–39.

Bertalanffy H, Eggert HR. Clinical long-term results of anterior discectomy without fusion for treatment of cervical radiculopathy and myelopathy. A follow-up of 164 cases. Acta Neurochir. 1988;90(3–4):127–35.

Borsari V, Fini M, Giavaresi G, et al. Sandblasted titanium osteointegration in young, aged and ovariectomized sheep. Int J Artif Organs. 2007;30(2):163–72.

Bryan Jr VE. Cervical motion segment replacement. Eur Spine J. 2002;11(Suppl 2):S92–7.

Cardoso MJ, Rosner MK. Multilevel cervical arthroplasty with artificial disc replacement. Neurosurg Focus. 2010;28(5):E19.

Caspar W, Barbier DD, Klara PM. Anterior cervical fusion and Caspar plate stabilization for cervical trauma. Neurosurgery. 1989;25(4):491–502.

Chen Y, Wang X, Lu X, et al. Comparison of titanium and polyetheretherketone (PEEK) cages in the surgical treatment of multilevel cervical spondylotic myelopathy: a prospective, randomized, control study with over 7-year follow-up. Eur Spine J. 2013;22(7):1539–46.

Cloward RB. The anterior approach for removal of ruptured cervical disks. J Neurosurg. 1958;15(6):602–17.

Epstein NE. Iliac crest autograft versus alternative constructs for anterior cervical spine surgery: pros, cons, and costs. Surg Neurol Int. 2012;3(Suppl 3):S143–56.

Goel VK, Faizan A, Palepu V, Bhattacharya S. Parameters that effect spine biomechanics following cervical disc replacement. Eur Spine J. 2012;21(Suppl 5):S688–99.

Hermann HD. Metal plate fixation after anterior fusion of unstable fraction of the cervical spine. Acta Neurochir. 1975;32:101–11.

Hong SW, Lee SH, Khoo LT, et al. A comparison of fixed-hole and slottedhole dynamic plates for anterior cervical discectomy and fusion. J Spinal Disord Tech. 2010;23(1):22–6.

Kim PK, Alexander JT. Indications for circumferential surgery for cervical spondylotic myelopathy. Spine J. 2006;6(6 Suppl):299S–307S.

Komotar RJ, Mocco J, Kaiser MG. Surgical management of cervical myelopathy: indications and techniques for laminectomy and fusion. Spine J. 2006;6(6 Suppl):252S–67S.

König SA, Spetzger U. Distractable titanium cages versus PEEK cages versus iliac crest bone grafts for the replacement of cervical vertebrae. Minim Invasive Ther Allied Technol. 2014;23(2):102–5.

König SA, Ranguis S, Spetzger U. Management of complex cervical instability. J Neurol Surg A Cent Eur Neurosurg. 2013;76(2):119–25. doi:10.1055/s–0033–1345095.

König SA, Ranguis C, Spetzger U. Hybrid Solutions for the Surgical Treatment of Multilevel Degenerative Cervical Disk Disease. Surg J 2015;1:e16–e22.

Le H, Thongtrangan I, Kim DH. Historical review of cervical arthroplasty. Neurosurg Focus. 2004;17(3):E1.

Medow JE, Trost G, Sandin J. Surgical management of cervical myelopathy: indications and techniques for surgical corpectomy. Spine J. 2006;6(6 Suppl):233S–41S.

Park SB, Jahng TA, Chung CK. Remodeling of adjacent spinal alignments following cervical arthroplasty and anterior discectomy and fusion. Eur Spine J. 2012;21(2):322–7.

Richards O, Choi D, Timothy J. Cervical arthroplasty: the beginning, the middle, the end? Br J Neurosurg. 2012;26(1):2–6.

Roosen K. Knochenzement als Ersatzmaterial für cervicale Bandscheiben. Fortschr Med. 1982;100(45):2120–6.

Shin DA, Yi S, Yoon do H, Kim KN, Shin HC. Artificial disc replacement combined with fusion versus two-level fusion in cervical two-level disc disease. Spine. 2009;34(11):1153–9.

Slivka MA, Spenciner DB, Seim HB, et al. High rate of fusion in sheep cervical spines following anterior interbody surgery with absorbable and nonabsorbable implant devices. Spine. 2006;31(24):2772–7.

Spetzger U, Schilling AV, Winkler G, Wahrburg J, König A. The past, present and future of minimally invasive spine surgery: a review and speculative outlook. Minim Invasive Ther Allied Technol. 2013;22(4):227–41.

Svedmark P, Lundh F, Németh G, et al. Motion analysis of total cervical disc replacements using computed tomography: preliminary experience with nine patients and a model. Acta Radiol. 2011;52(10):1128–37.

Surgical Technique

8

The anterior standard approach is the most frequently used surgical approach to the cervical spine. It is suitable for discectomy as well as for corpectomy with anterior plating. The posterior approach allows laminectomy and fusion as well as open-door laminoplasty. When performing the anterior approach, it is possible to use anatomical landmarks (hyoid bone, thyroid cartilage, tuberculum caroticum) already when starting with the skin incision. During the posterior approach, it is only possible to identify the midline with the help of the spinous processes. The spinous processes of C2 and C7 are usually longer than the spinous processes of C3 to C6; thus, they can be used as anatomical landmarks.

8.1 Anterior Approach, Discectomy, Cage Implantation and Total Disc Replacement

8.1.1 Anterior Approach to the Cervical Spine and Discectomy

The operation is performed in supine position with the head in a slightly extended position. By adjusting the operating table, the patient's head should be placed higher than the heart to avoid venous congestion and thus increased venous bleeding in the spinal canal during surgery. A fluoroscope is integrated in the operative setup and covered with sterile drapes.

The skin incision starts in the midline and is about 4 cm long (Fig. 8.1). It should be placed in a skinfold to achieve an optimum cosmetic result after surgery. When performing multilevel surgery (three or more levels), most surgeons prefer a longitudinal incision over the anterior edge of the sternocleidomastoid muscle. In case of good anatomical conditions, it is possible to use the transverse standard incision for three-level surgery as well.

It is possible to identify certain cervical levels by anatomical landmarks before the skin incision:

A. König, U. Spetzger, *Degenerative Diseases of the Cervical Spine*,
DOI 10.1007/978-3-319-47298-0_8

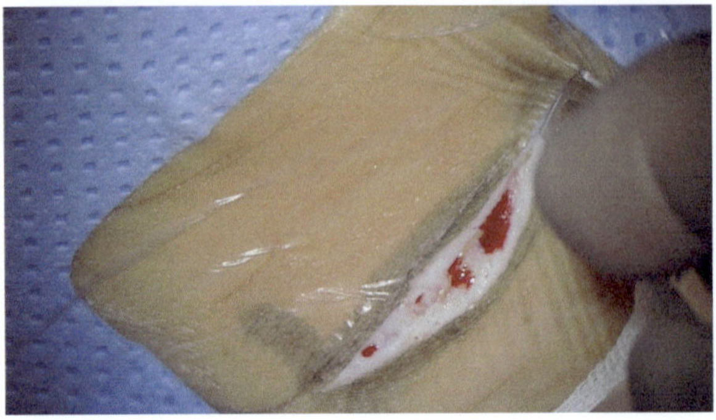

Fig. 8.1 Skin incision for an anterior approach to C4/5

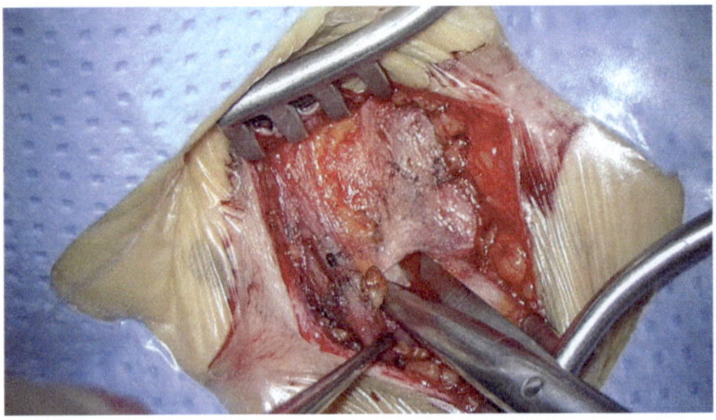

Fig. 8.2 Incision of the platysma

- C2/3: mandibular angle
- C3/4: hyoid bone
- C4/5: upper edge of the thyroid cartilage
- C5/6: lower edge of the thyroid cartilage
- C6/7: middle between lower edge of the thyroid cartilage and sternum

After dissection and incision of the platysma, the superficial fascia is dissected and incised medially to the sternocleidomastoid muscle (Figs. 8.2, 8.3 and 8.4). Afterwards the common carotid artery is identified by using blunt dissection of the straight cervical muscles (Figs. 8.5 and 8.6). Then the neurovascular bundle of the neck (common carotid artery, internal jugular vein, vagus nerve) is lateralised. Finally, the hypopharynx (above C5) or the trachea and oesophagus, respectively, are medialised (Fig. 8.7). After the visualisation of the anterior aspect of the cervical spine, the prevertebral fascia is incised and dissected. For identification of the level C5/6, palpation of the tuberculum caroticum is helpful (Fig. 2.2).

The surgical field is exhibited by self-holding soft tissue retractors (Fig. 8.9). Afterwards the identification of the right level is verified using a fluoroscope. Then, Caspar pins (Caspar et al. 1989) are screwed into the vertebral bodies of the affected level (Fig. 8.10 and 8.11). This step is also checked with the fluoroscope. Afterwards the distractor is put on the pins and fixed. A slight distraction is applied until the anterior longitudinal ligament is tensed (Fig. 8.12).

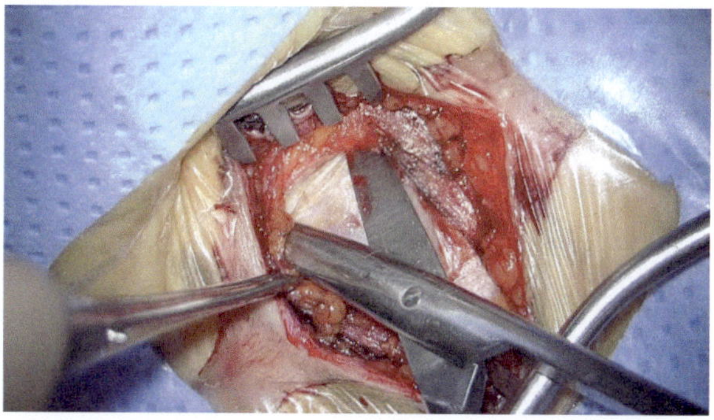

Fig. 8.3 Exposure of the superficial fascia

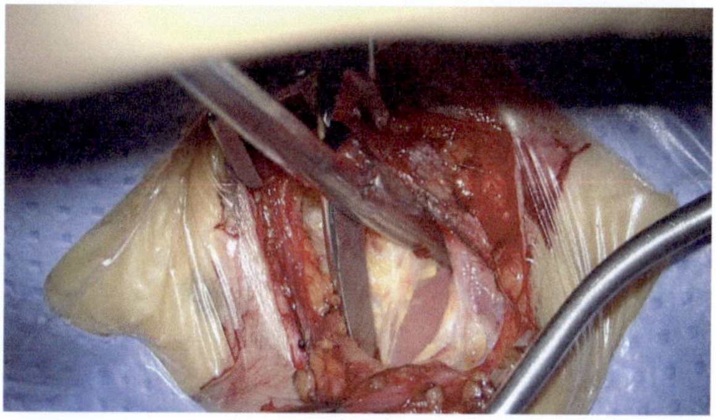

Fig. 8.4 Incision of the superficial fascia

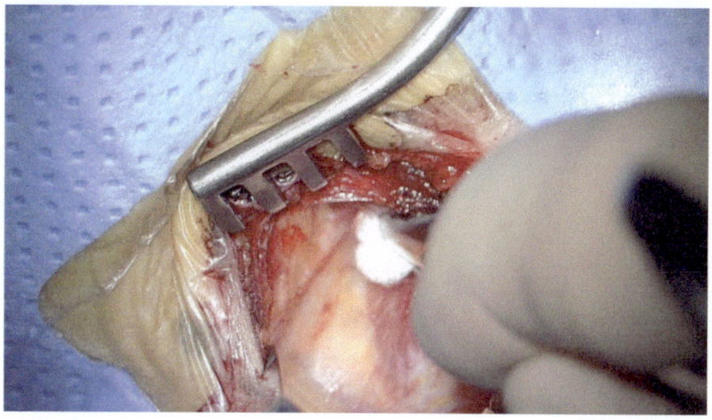

Fig. 8.5 Medialising of the straight cervical muscles

Under microscopic view, the anterior longitudinal ligament is incised and resected (Fig. 8.13). Now, loose disc material can be removed with a forceps (Fig. 8.14). The discectomy is completed with a sharp spoon. During this process, remnants of the disc as well as the hyaline cartilage are removed from the endplates without perforating the bony endplates of the adjacent vertebrae (Fig. 8.15).

The resection of posterior osteophytes and the microsurgical decompression of the spinal cord can be achieved by using either a Kerrison punch or a high-speed drill (Fig. 8.16). When using a fluted ball tool with the drilling system, the resection of osteophytes can be done fast, but there is a higher risk for injuring the dural or even the spinal cord. Therefore, this option should be chosen by very experienced

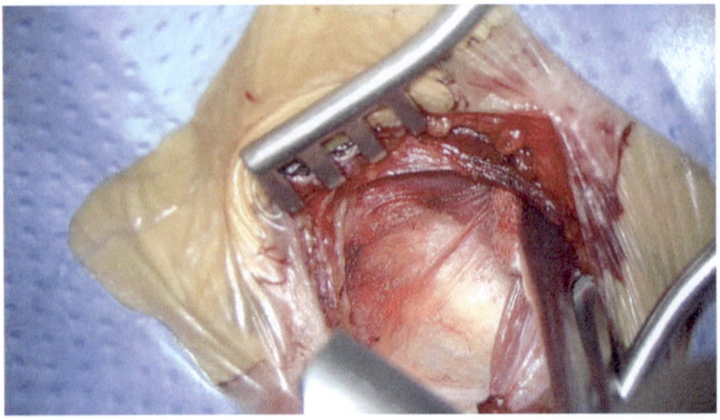

Fig. 8.6 Exposure of the common carotid artery

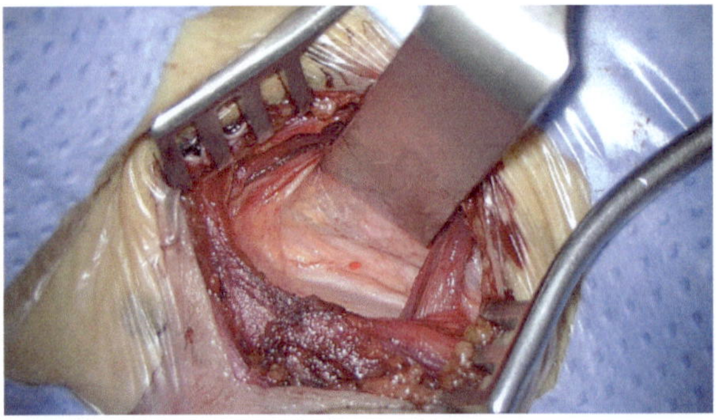

Fig. 8.7 Medialising of the hypopharynx

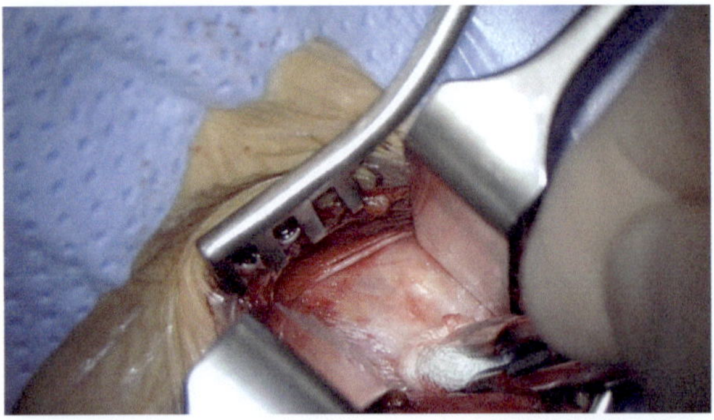

Fig. 8.8 Exposure of the ventral surface of the cervical spine

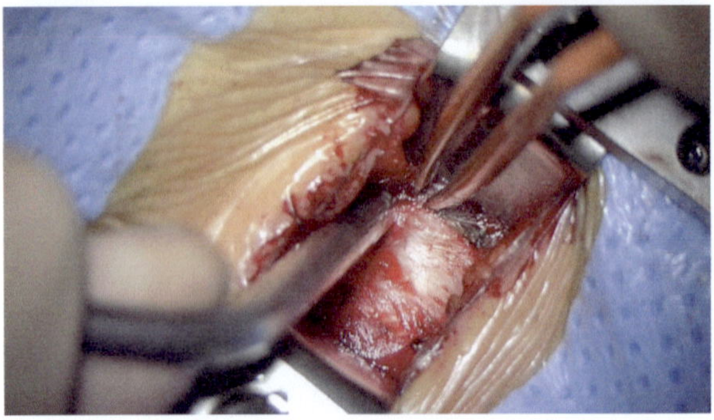

Fig. 8.9 Self-holding soft tissue retractor

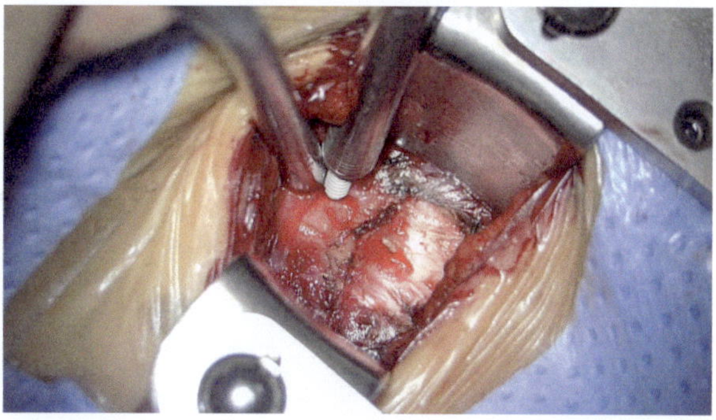

Fig. 8.10 Screwing in a Caspar pin into the superior vertebral body

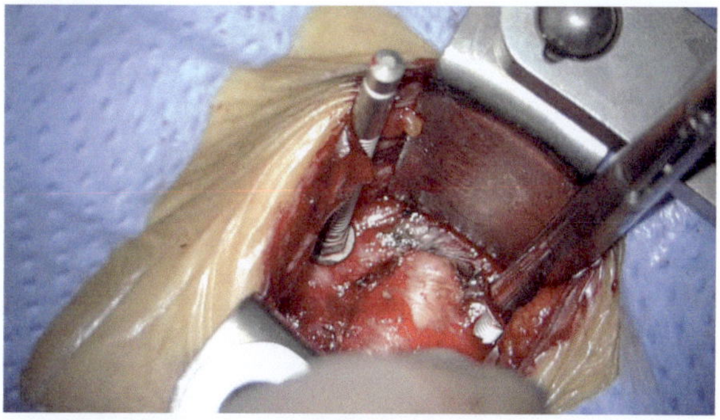

Fig. 8.11 Screwing in a Caspar pin into the inferior vertebral body

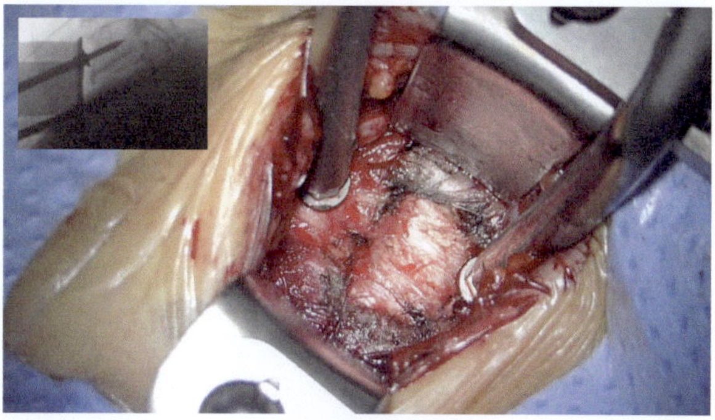

Fig. 8.12 Introducing of the Caspar distractor. Small image: fluoroscopic image of the Caspar pins, lateral view

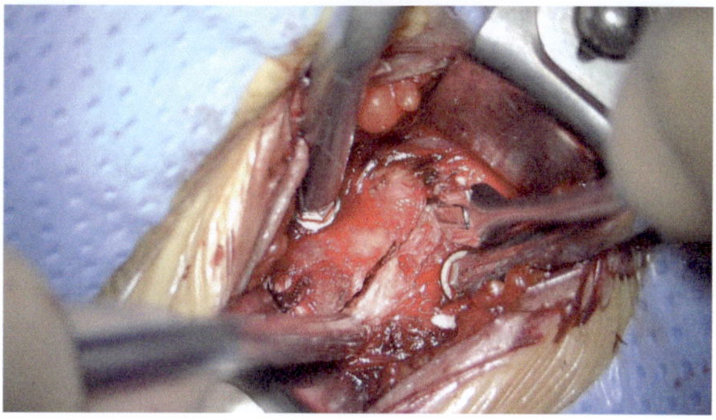

Fig. 8.13 Incision of the anterior longitudinal ligament at the height of the intervertebral disc

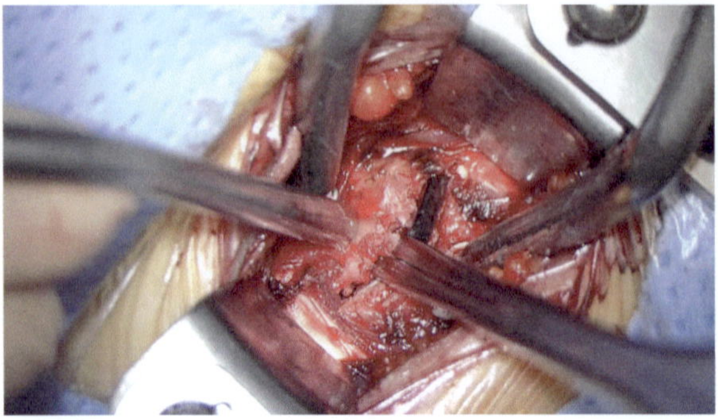

Fig. 8.14 Start of the discectomy with a forceps

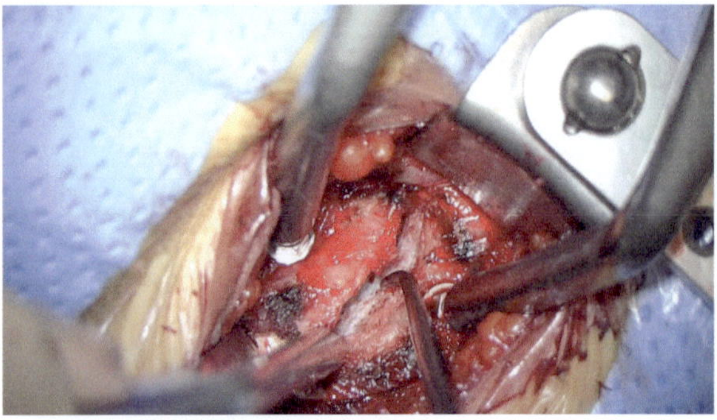

Fig. 8.15 Completion of the discectomy with a sharp spoon

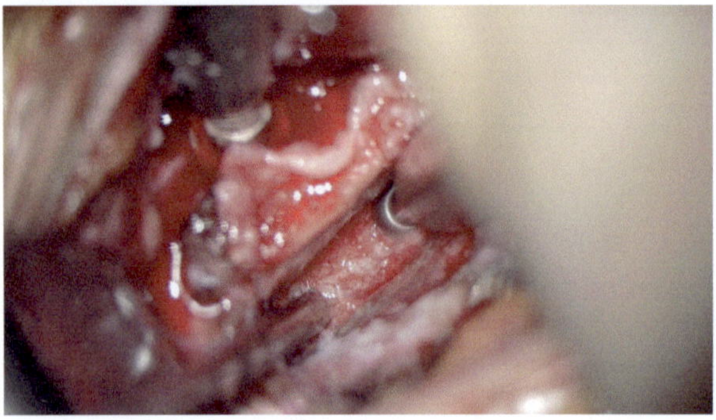

Fig. 8.16 Resection of posterior osteophytes with a diamond drill

surgeons only. Using a diamond drill is an alternative with a lower risk of dural injury, but the higher temperature during the drilling procedure has to be taken into account. When using a diamond drill, it is crucial to use enough irrigation and to interrupt drilling from time to time to avoid thermal damage of neural structures. The resection of osteophytes by drilling increases the likelihood of heterotope ossification and consecutive bony bridging of the treated level. This fact has to be taken into account when implanting a prosthesis.

Afterwards the posterior longitudinal ligament is perforated with a filigree nerve hook and resected with a 2-mm Kerrison punch (Fig. 8.17). By doing so the spinal canal is decompressed step by step since it is possible to resect thickened ligaments

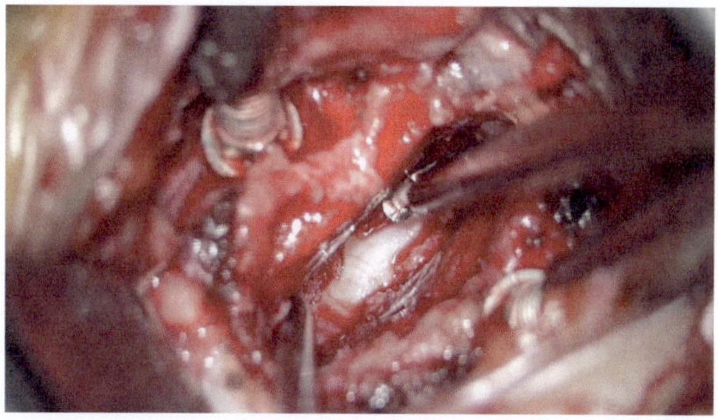

Fig. 8.17 Resection of the posterior longitudinal ligament with a Kerrison punch

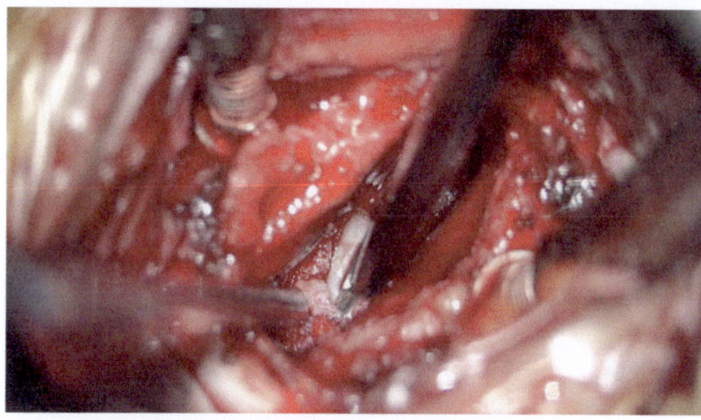

Fig. 8.18 Decompression of the right neuroforamen with a Kerrison punch

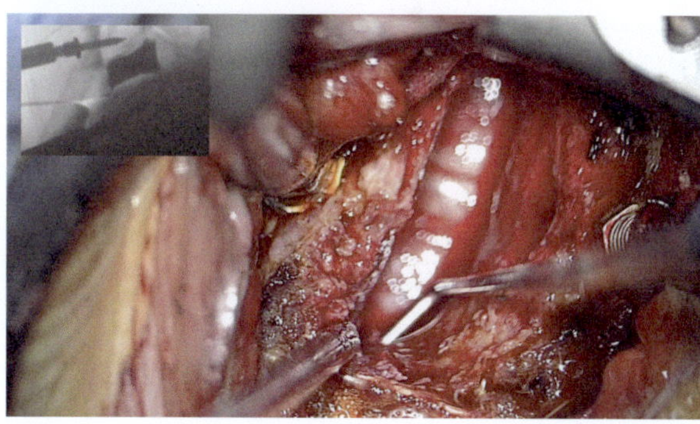

Fig. 8.19 Checking the decompression with a nerve hook. Small image: lateral fluoroscopy after application of contrast agent into the intervertebral disc space

and bone behind vertebral bodies and in the neuroforamina (Fig. 8.18). The decompression is checked under fluoroscopy with a nerve hook (Fig. 8.19). When using the Kerrison punch for resection of posterior osteophytes, it is crucial to bear in mind that this leads to an additional space occupation by the instrument with consecutive worsening of a pre-existing myelopathy. Compared to drilling, the use of the Kerrison punch is a bit more time-consuming, and it has the potential disadvantage of venous bleedings from cancellous bone that can be stopped by the heat resulting from using a diamond drill.

After the resection of the posterior longitudinal ligament and posterior osteophytes, the distraction of the vertebral bodies is slightly increased, and the trial head of the cage or prosthesis is inserted to determine the size of the definite implant (Fig. 8.20). Finally, the implant is inserted and the distraction is taken away (Fig. 8.21). Before that, the effect of the decompression and the right depth of the implant can be assessed by application of a contrast agent into the intervertebral disc space and the epidural space, respectively (Fig. 8.22). Afterwards, the wound is closed layer by layer.

8.1.2 Implantation of an Intervertebral Cage

The implantation of a cage is usually an uncomplicated procedure. Despite the numerous models of cages on the market, the basic surgical steps of implantation are the same. After discectomy (see Sect. 8.1.1), the size of the cage is determined by inserting a trial head into the disc space (Fig. 8.23). In most cases, the height of the cage varies between 4 and 5 mm, the width varies between 16 and 20 mm, and the depth varies between 12 and 16 mm. It is recommended to use a cage model where the instruments for insertion have a stop device (see Sect. 10.4). This increases safety during insertion of trial head and cage, especially when it is necessary to use a hammer. Without a stop device, the risk of accidental injury of the spinal cord is much higher, especially during educational surgeries.

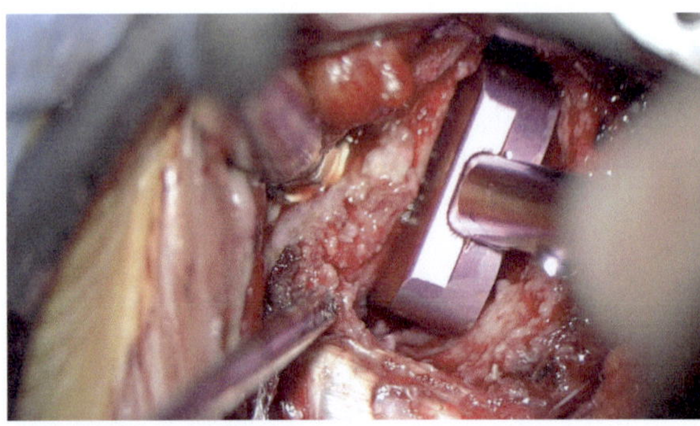

Fig. 8.20 Insertion of the trial head to determine the size of the final implant

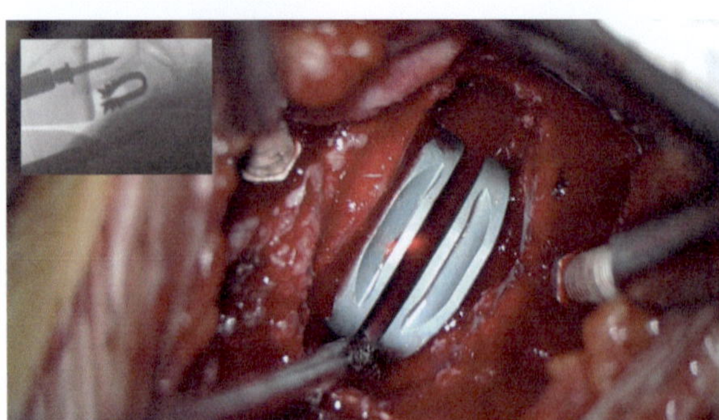

Fig. 8.21 Implantation of a dynamic cervical implant DCI™. Small image: lateral fluoroscopic view of the implant

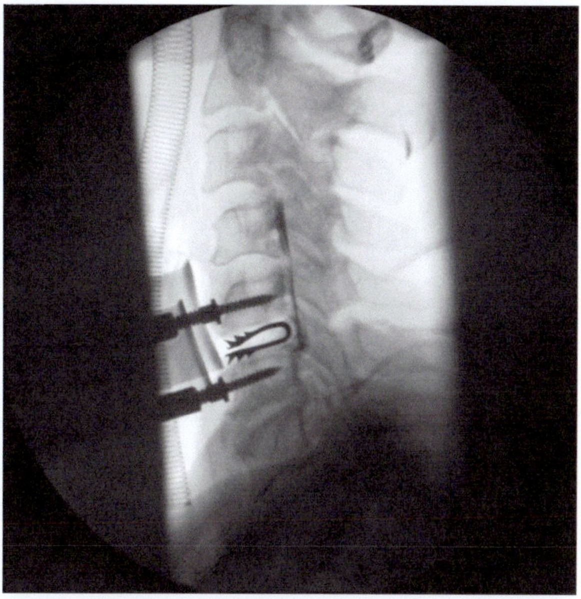

Fig. 8.22 Fluoroscopic image after implantation of a DCI™ with epidural application of contrast agent (to be seen behind the vertebral bodies of C3, C4 and partially C5) to check the adequate depth of the implant

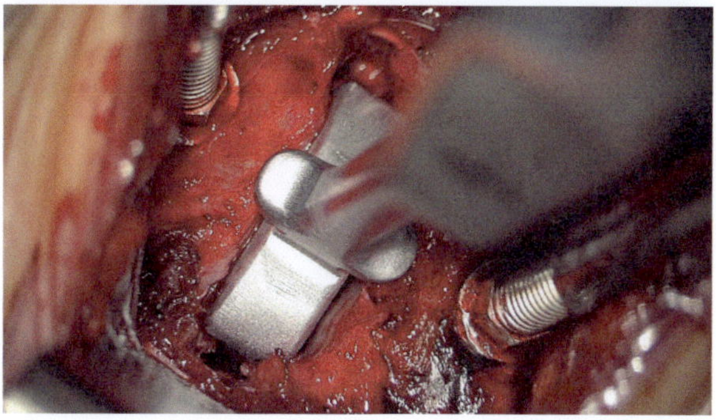

Fig. 8.23 Insertion of a trial implant (4 × 16 × 14 mm) for measuring the dimensions of the disc space

To achieve a safe bony fusion of the adjacent vertebral bodies after 3 months, it is helpful to fill the cage with osteoinductive material, especially when using PEEK cages (Fig. 8.24). The anchorage of the cage in the endplates is achieved by small spikes on the surface of the cage and the profile of the surface itself (Fig. 8.25). The insertion of the implant is done under lateral fluoroscopy and after temporary increase of distraction. After taking back distraction, the adequate position is finally checked and documented by fluoroscopy.

8.1.3 Total Disc Replacement

During total disc replacement, the height, width and depth of the final implant are also determined with a trial implant. Depending on the model, the endplates of the vertebral bodies have to be prepared with special chisels. For example, the

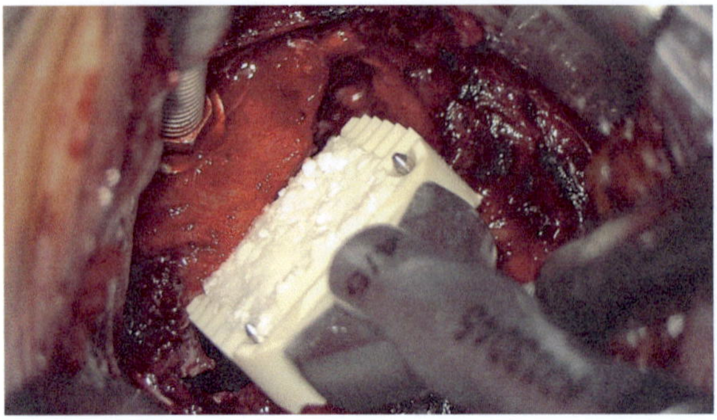

Fig. 8.24 Implantation of a PEEK cage Cornerstone TM (Medtronic, Meerbusch, Germany) filled with osteoinductive Material (Vitoss TM by Stryker, Duisburg, Germany)

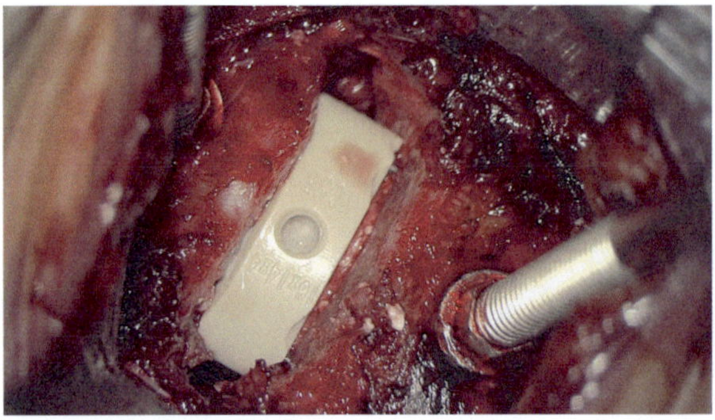

Fig. 8.25 Final position of the cage

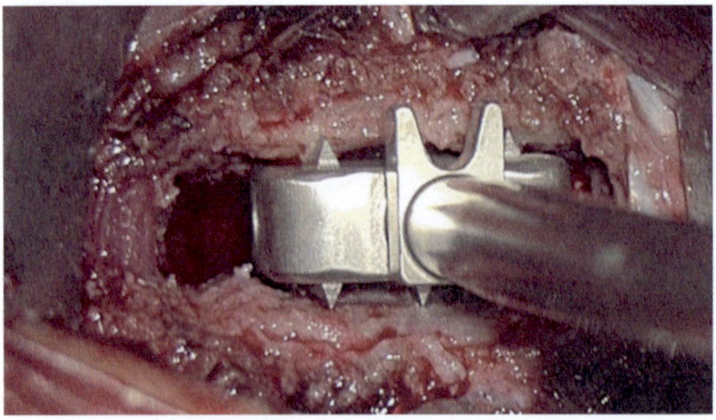

Fig. 8.26 Chisel for the preparation of keels for the M6C prosthesis. At the upper edge of the instrument, a stop device avoids the chisel to slide too deep into the disc space

implantation of an M6C prosthesis (Spinal Kinetics, Sunnyvale, CA, USA) requires preparation of the endplates with a chisel with three keels that create three tracks for the anchorage of the implant (Fig. 8.26). The M6C chisel has stop device to avoid accidental injury of the spinal cord (Fig. 8.26).

After preparing the endplates, it is crucial to remove remnants of the bone and cartilage (Fig. 8.27). If endplate preparation is consequently done in the midline, the implant will be strictly positioned in the midline, too (Fig. 8.28).

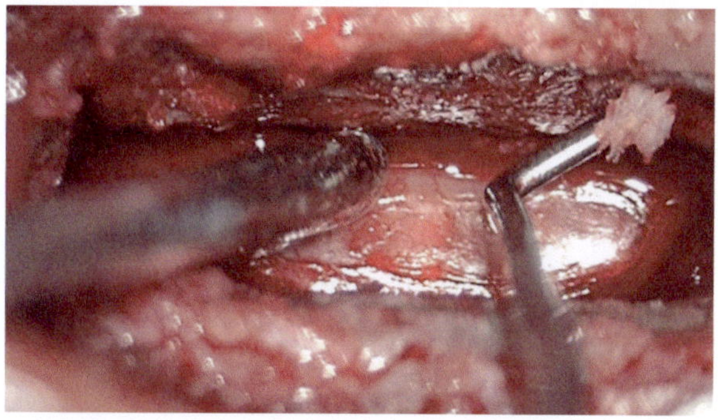

Fig. 8.27 Removal of bony and cartilaginous remnants after preparation of the endplates to avoid dislocation of these remnants with the consequence of compression of neural structures

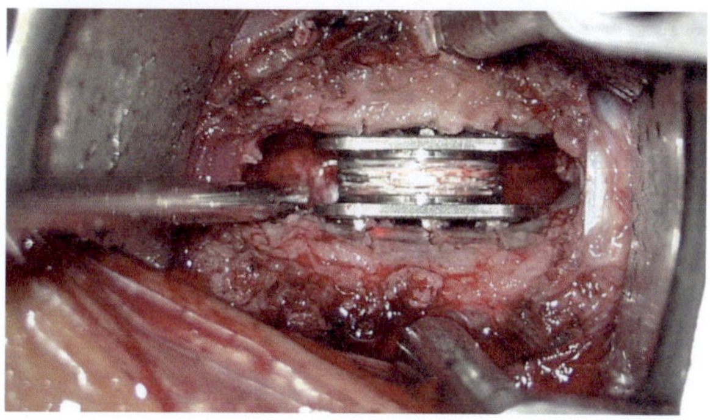

Fig. 8.28 Final position of the M6C prosthesis in the intervertebral disc space. Anchorage of the implant in the endplates with keels. Due to the far lateral dissection of the uncinated recesses, both neuroforamina can be seen even after TDR

8.2 Corpectomy and Anterior Plating

The surgical approach for corpectomy and anterior plating is the anterolateral standard approach in supine position as it is described in Sect. 8.1.1. Under slight distraction and microscopical view, a discectomy of the adjacent intervertebral discs is performed (Figs. 8.29, 8.30 and 8.31). During corpectomy, it is crucial to remove the cartilage of the endplates as described for discectomy to enable secondary bony fusion. The surgeon has to avoid injury of the cortical bone of the adjacent vertebral bodies because they provide load bearing and stability.

Corpectomy is usually done using a high-speed drill (Fig. 8.31). Alternatively, a rongeur or Kerrison punch can be used for corpectomy. The posterior wall of the vertebral body can be safely removed with a diamond drill (Fig. 8.32). Posterior osteophytes can be removed with a diamond drill, too, or with a Kerrison punch when resecting the posterior longitudinal ligament (Figs. 8.32 and 8.33). For the resection of the posterior longitudinal ligament, it is crucial to use a Kerrison punch with a thin footplate to avoid surgical morbidity of the spinal cord (Figs. 8.34 and 8.35). After completing the decompression of the spinal canal, the height of the corpectomy defect is measured to determine the height of the vertebral body replacement. Afterwards an autologous iliac crest bone graft is harvested or the surgeon chooses an implant made of titanium or PEEK (Medow et al. 2006; König et al.

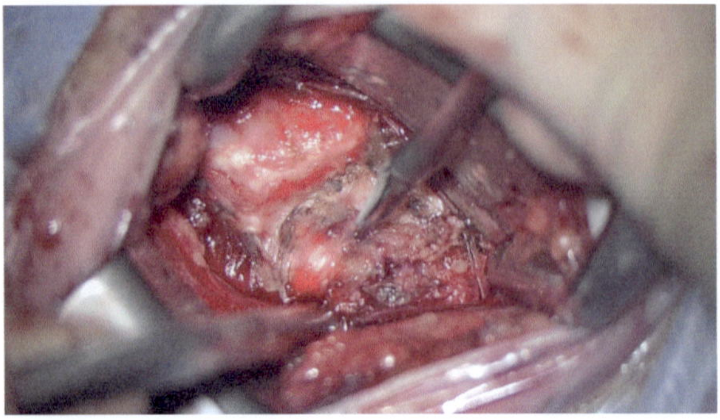

Fig. 8.29 Incision of the anterior longitudinal ligament at the height of the intervertebral disc adjacent to the vertebral body that has to be removed

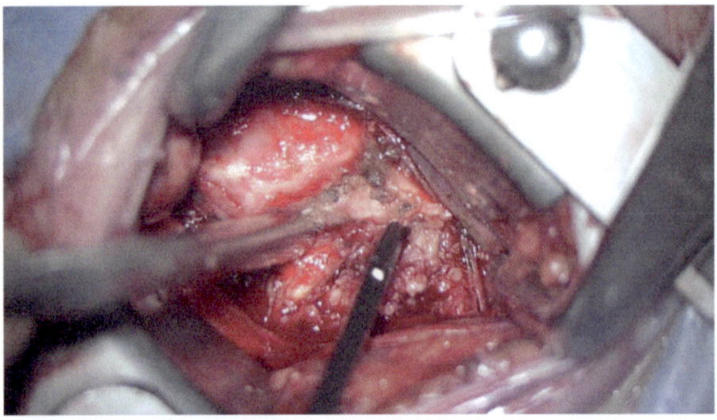

Fig. 8.30 Discectomy with a disc forceps

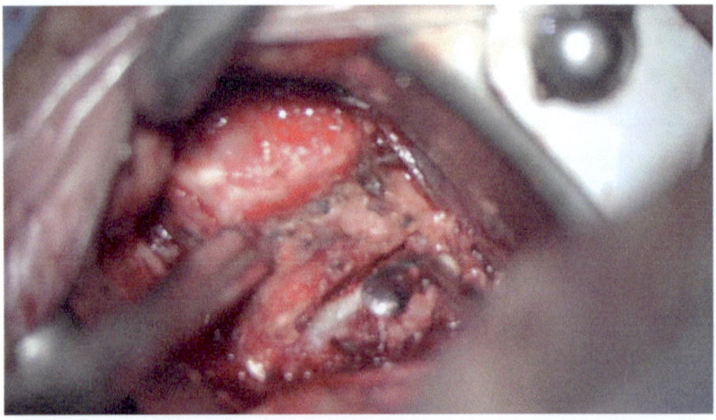

Fig. 8.31 Removal of hyaline cartilage at the endplates with a sharp spoon

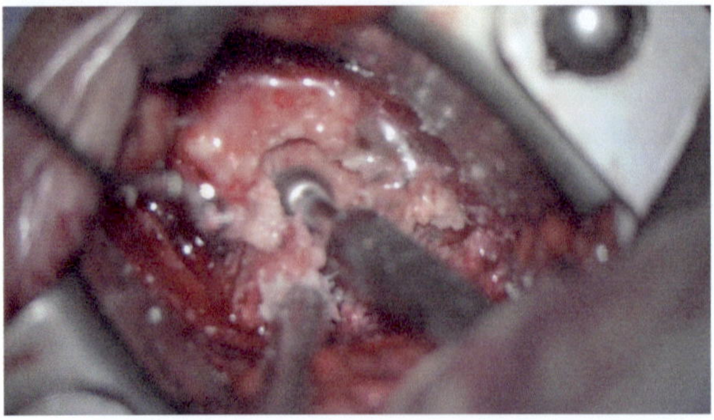

Fig. 8.32 Removal of the vertebral body with a high-speed drill

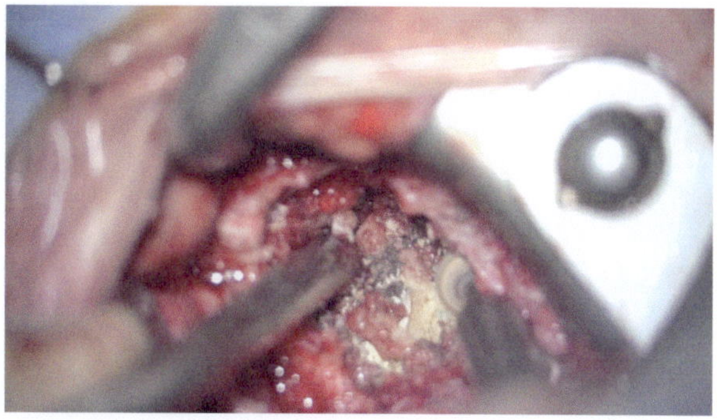

Fig. 8.33 Removal of the posterior wall of the vertebral body with a high-speed diamond drill

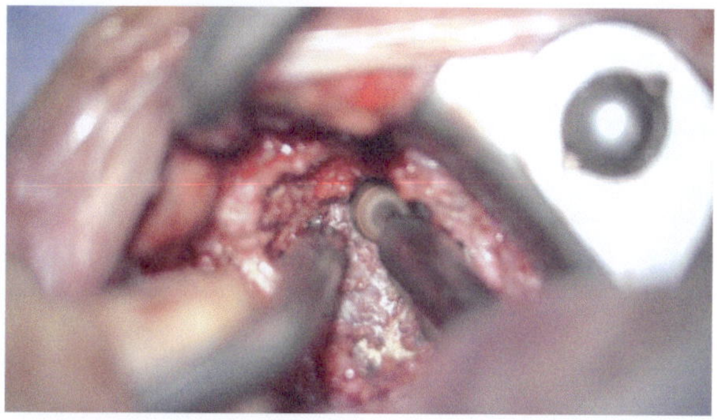

Fig. 8.34 Removal of posterior osteophytes with a high-speed diamond drill

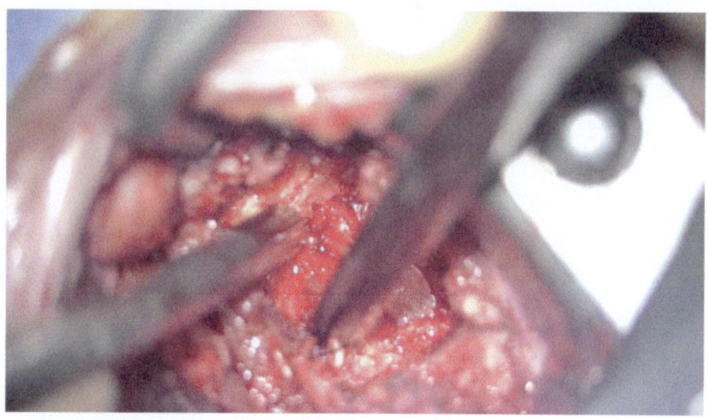

Fig. 8.35 Decompression of the spinal canal by resecting the posterior longitudinal ligament with a Kerrison punch

2013). After implanting, the vertebral body replacement distraction is taken away, and thus the implant is fixed due to axial pressure (Fig. 8.36).

After removal of the Caspar pins anterior fusion by plating osteosynthesis is performed (Figs. 8.37, 8.38, 8.39 and 8.40). The length of the vertebral body screws has to be measured preoperatively using the patient's CT scans. In most cases, the length of the screws is between 14 and 20 mm. Furthermore, the surgeon has to decide if monocortical or bicortical screwing is aimed. The autologous iliac crest bone craft has to be fixed with shorter screws (10–12 mm) since it has a smaller depth compared to vertebral bodies. When screws are placed into the bone graft, it is crucial to avoid secondary dislocation of the graft and consecutive compression of the spinal cord.

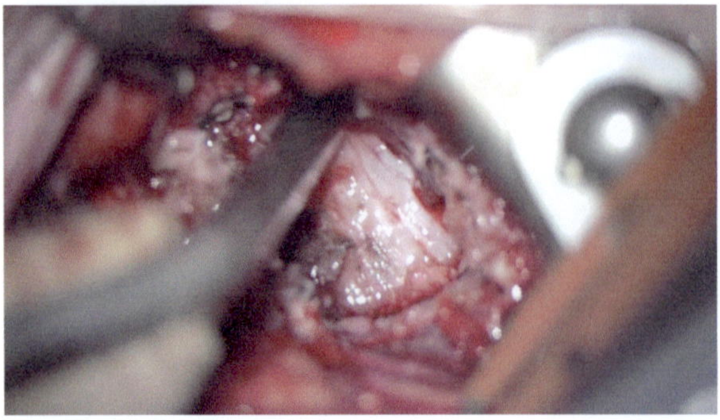

Fig. 8.36 Exposure of the dura of the cervical spinal cord during decompression

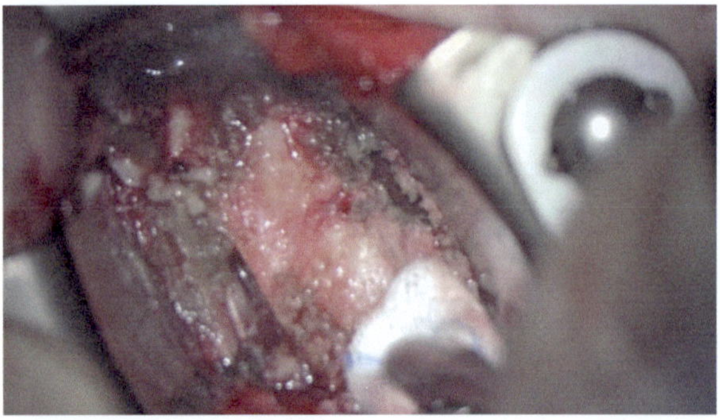

Fig. 8.37 Insertion of the iliac crest bone graft into the corpectomy defect

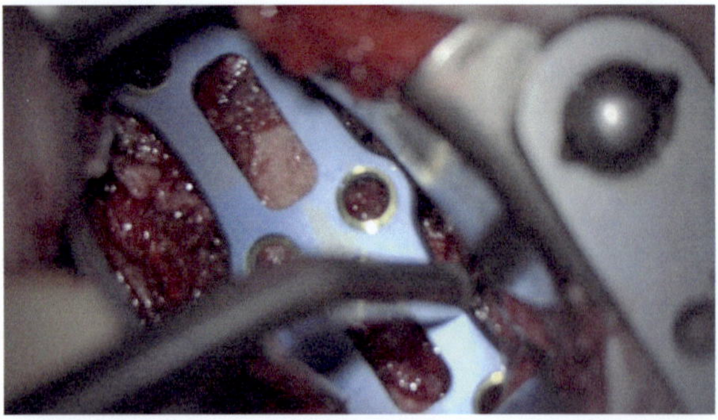

Fig. 8.38 Placement of the anterior plate (Reflex Hybrid by Stryker, Duisburg, Germany). In the holes in the middle the locking rings can be seen which provide locking when tightening the screws

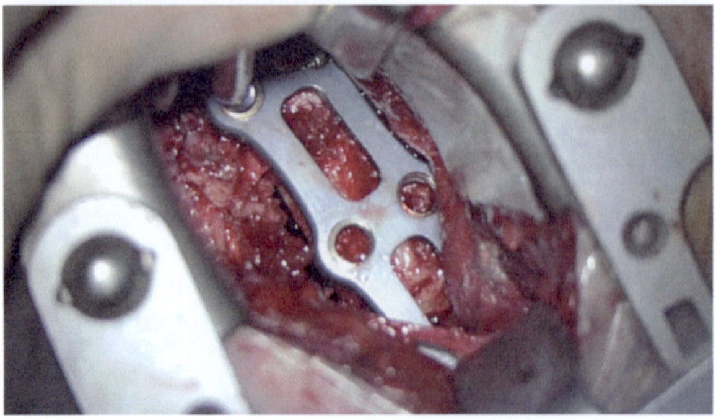

Fig. 8.39 Placement of self-drilling screws for fixation of the plate to vertebra C4

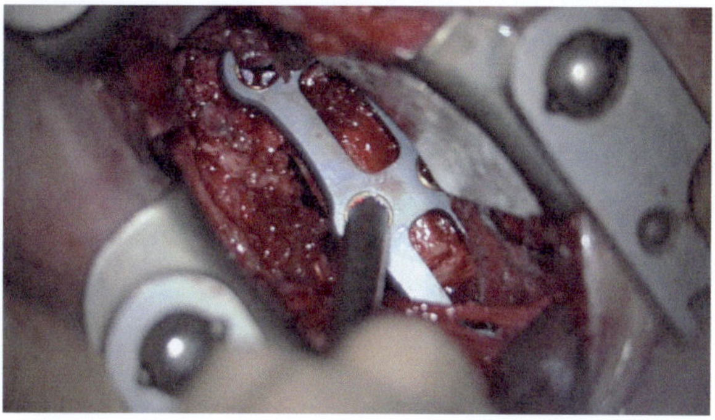

Fig. 8.40 Fixing the plate to the iliac crest bone graft. It is crucial to avoid secondary dislocation of the bone graft and to use shorter screws compared to the vertebral bodies for avoiding pressure to the spinal cord

As described in Sect. 7.2.2, there are different options of angle variability or angle stability of the screws depending on the manufacturer of the system. Often there is a blocking mechanism or a special instrument providing a certain angle of convergence in the axial plane to avoid injury of the vertebral artery by misplaced screws. Most manufacturers offer self-drilling screws that can be placed without pre-drilling under fluoroscopic control. When all of the screws are finally tightened, they are locked by a blocking mechanism within the plate (e.g. reflex hybrid, Fig. 8.38) or by additional small locking screws (e.g. skyline, Fig. 7.21).

8.3 Laminectomy and Posterior Fusion

The posterior approach is performed in prone position with the head fixed in the Mayfield clamp. After dissection of the insertions of the neck muscles in the midline, the laminae of the cervical vertebrae are exposed. The muscles have to be retracted as far as necessary to identify the lateral masses for the placement of screws under lateral fluoroscopy (Figs. 8.41 and 8.43). The direction of drilling the lateral masses was defined by Magerl as 25 degrees in lateral and 45 degrees in cranial direction (Komotar et al. 2006).

Afterwards the drill holes are checked with a probe to figure out if it is completely surrounded by the bone and if the hole is perforated in the anterior direction (Fig. 8.42). Furthermore, the depth of the drill holes is checked to find the adequate length for the lateral mass screws. The standard dimensions for lateral mass screws are a diameter of 3.5 mm and a length of 10–16 mm. When using screws that are too long, there is a potential risk of injuring the vertebral artery if the trajectory of drill hole is too far medially (Fig. 8.43).

When all screws are in place, the length of the connecting rods is measured (Fig. 8.44). In top loading systems like the Synapse system (Sect. 7.3.1), the polyaxiality of the screw heads is 50 degrees. Thus, it is usually quite easy to place the connecting rods into the screw heads. After tightening the locking screws, a transverse connector is added to increase stability of the whole construct (Fig. 8.45).

After completing the osteosynthesis, there is usually enough space to perform a laminectomy for decompression of the spinal canal (Fig. 8.46). Doing the

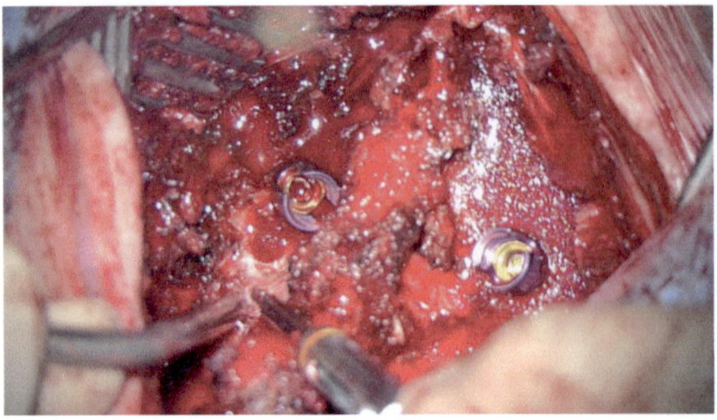

Fig. 8.41 Drilling holes for the lateral mass screws (diameter of the drill: 2.6 mm)

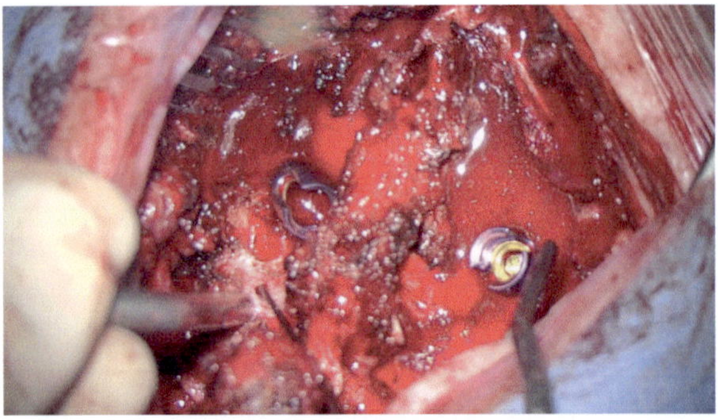

Fig. 8.42 Checking of the drill hole with a probe

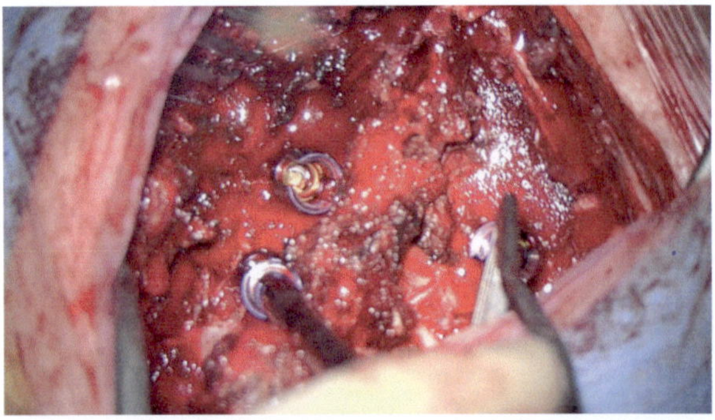

Fig. 8.43 Placement of a lateral mass screw

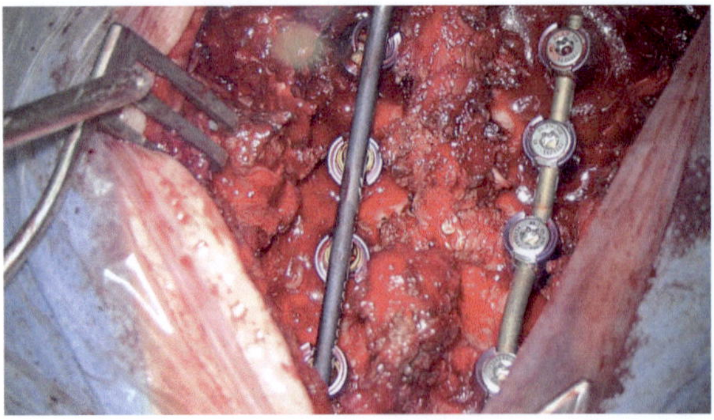

Fig. 8.44 Measuring the length of the connecting rod

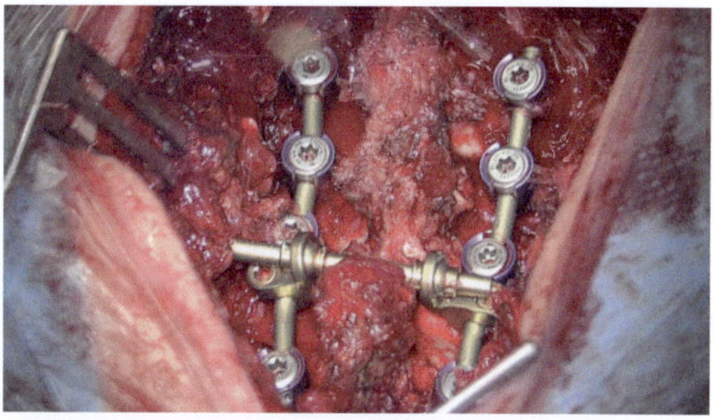

Fig. 8.45 Completed posterior instrumentation with transverse connector

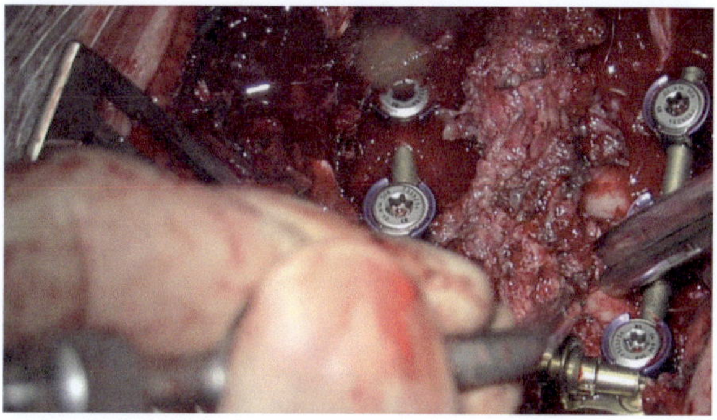

Fig. 8.46 Laminectomy with a Kerrison punch for decompression

laminectomy after finishing, the instrumentation eliminates the risk of accidental injury of the spinal cord by the screwdriver.

8.4 Open-Door Laminoplasty, Laminotomy, Foraminotomy and Modifications

8.4.1 Open-Door Laminoplasty

When using the classical technique, the laminae of usually three vertebrae are cut through at the transition of the lamina to the lateral mass with a craniotome or a jigsaw. On the opposite side, only a notch is drilled with a small diamond drill into the outer cortical bone to create a 'hinge' for the open 'door'. The opened laminae are fixed with titanium mini plates to the lateral masses to keep the widening of the spinal canal. A possible disadvantage of the classical technique is that a sufficient osteoligamentous decompression of the neuroforamen on the 'hinge' side is sometimes hard to achieve without compressing the spinal cord with the Kerrison punch. Therefore, the authors use a modified technique with a temporary laminectomy with a craniotome (Figs. 8.47, 8.48, 8.49, 8.50, 8.51, 8.52, 8.53 and 8.54). By using this technique, it is easy to decompress the lateral spinal canal on both sides. Furthermore, it is possible to decompress the spinal cord under the adjacent laminae by using an undercutting technique (König and Spetzger 2014a, b). After removing the laminae, they are liberated from remnants of the ligamenta flava to achieve an optimum

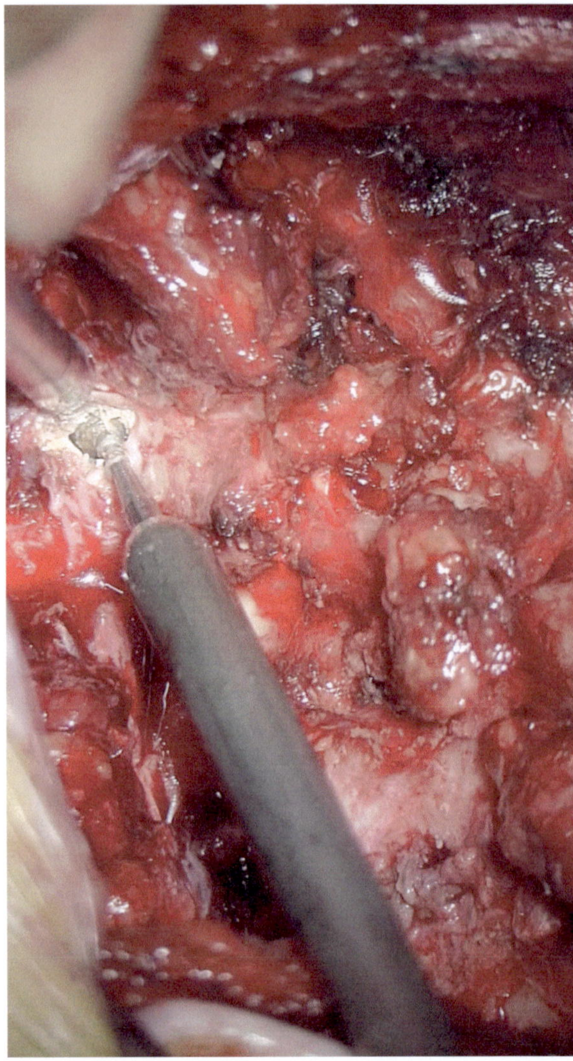

Fig. 8.47 Circumscribed laminotomy with a diamond drill as an entry for the craniotome

decompression of the spinal canal. Afterwards the laminae are pre-plated with titanium mini plates outside of the surgical field to eliminate the risk of spinal cord injury during screwing. Then the laminae are reinserted into the defect, and they are fixed asymmetrically with short plates on one side and longer plates on the other side (Fig. 8.55). Direct contact of the bone on the short side promotes bony healing. The described technique is a laminoplasty in the narrower sense.

8.4.2 Laminotomy and Foraminotomy

In cases of circumscribed stenoses, it is possible to create a longitudinal oval interlaminar opening (partial hemilaminectomy of two adjacent laminae) with a

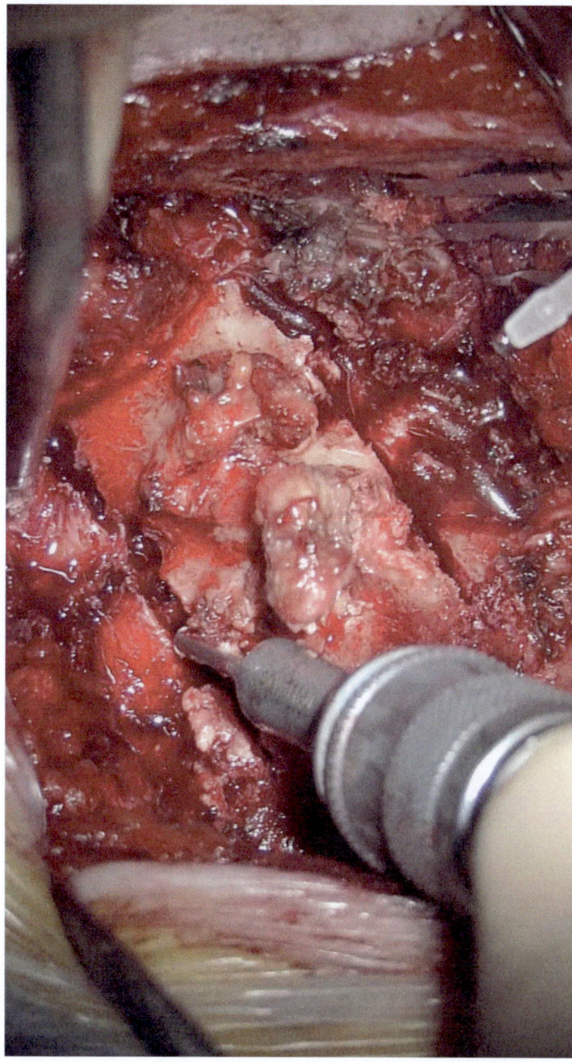

Fig. 8.48 Cut through the laminae on the left side with a craniotome

diamond drill under microscopic view. This procedure is adequate for unilateral posterior ligamentous hypertrophy and avoids a complete hemilaminectomy or laminectomy.

For the special case of a far lateral disc herniation or a circumscribed stenosis of the neuroforamen, it is possible to perform a foraminotomy as described by Frykholm. After a paramedian skin incision, an extra small retractor (Piccolino™ by Medicon, Tuttlingen, Germany) is centred over the transition from two adjacent laminae to the facet joint. After fluoroscopic control of the approach, a minimal lateral laminotomy is created with a small diamond drill and a 2-mm Kerrison punch with exposure of the proximal nerve root (Fig. 8.56). By using the undercutting technique, the foramen is decompressed distally. If necessary, a disc sequestrum can be removed with a nerve hook. This technique is most suitable for the

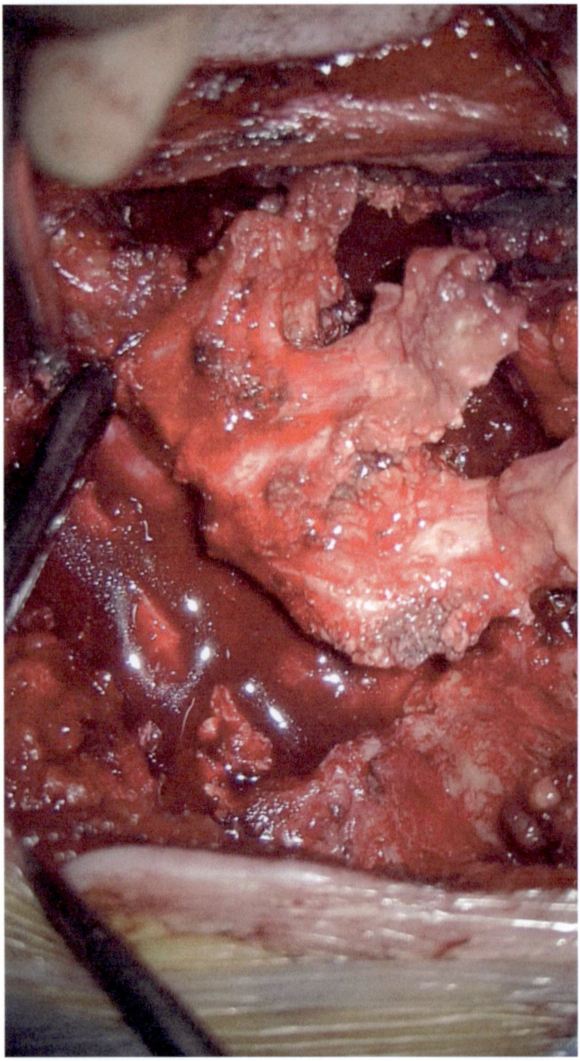

Fig. 8.49 Elevation of the complex consisting of laminae, spinous processes, ligamenta flava and interspinous ligaments

levels C6/7 and C7/T1 since fluoroscopy is sometimes difficult at these levels during the anterior approach due to high shoulders.

8.5 Combined Approach

If a combined approach is indicated (corpectomy of two or more levels, poor bone quality, etc.), it should be done as a single-stage procedure to avoid a second intubation and anaesthesia as well as to minimise operation time and blood loss (Kim and Alexander 2006; König et al. 2013; König and Spetzger 2014a, b). Furthermore, the hospital stay is shortened.

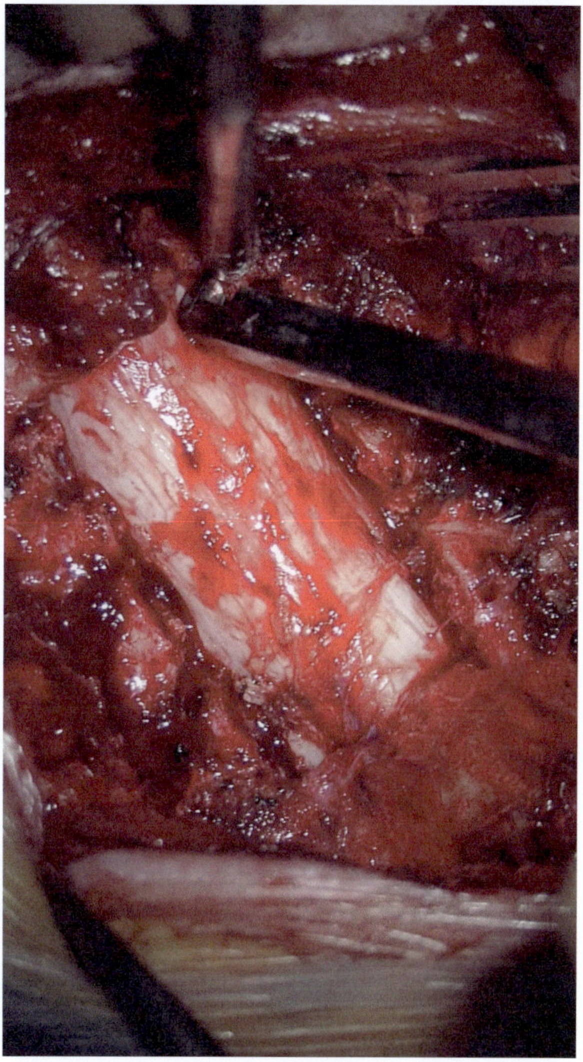

Fig. 8.50 Posterior decompression with a Kerrison punch

The surgical technique of a single-stage combined approach and fusion accords to the description of anterior technique (Sect. 8.2) and posterior technique (Sect. 8.3). The surgery usually starts with discectomy/corpectomy and continues with posterior instrumentation after changing the patient's position, whereas anterior decompression is often sufficient, and thus, posterior decompression by laminectomy is only necessary in selected cases.

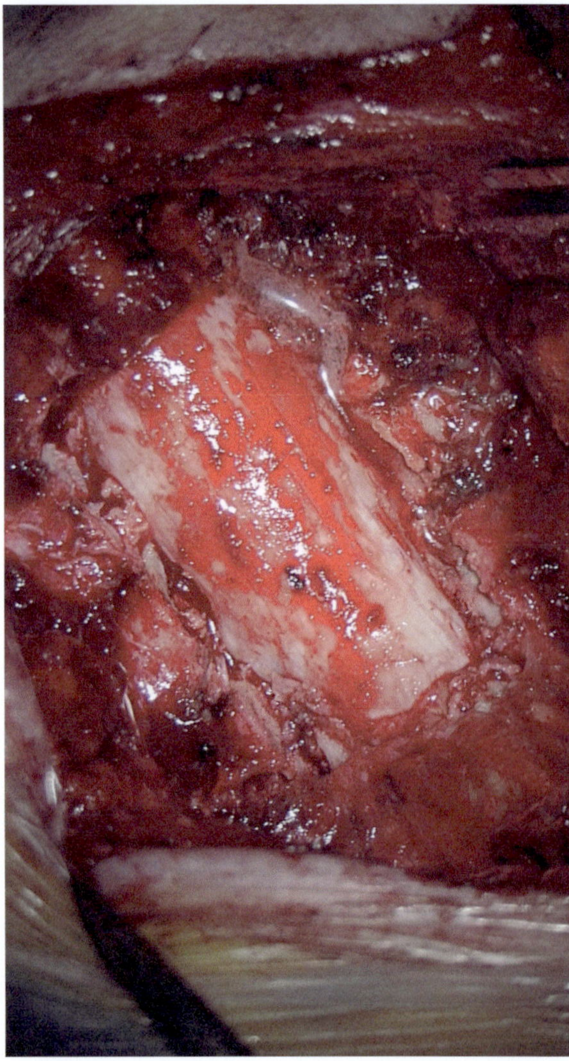

Fig. 8.51 Completed decompression of the spinal canal

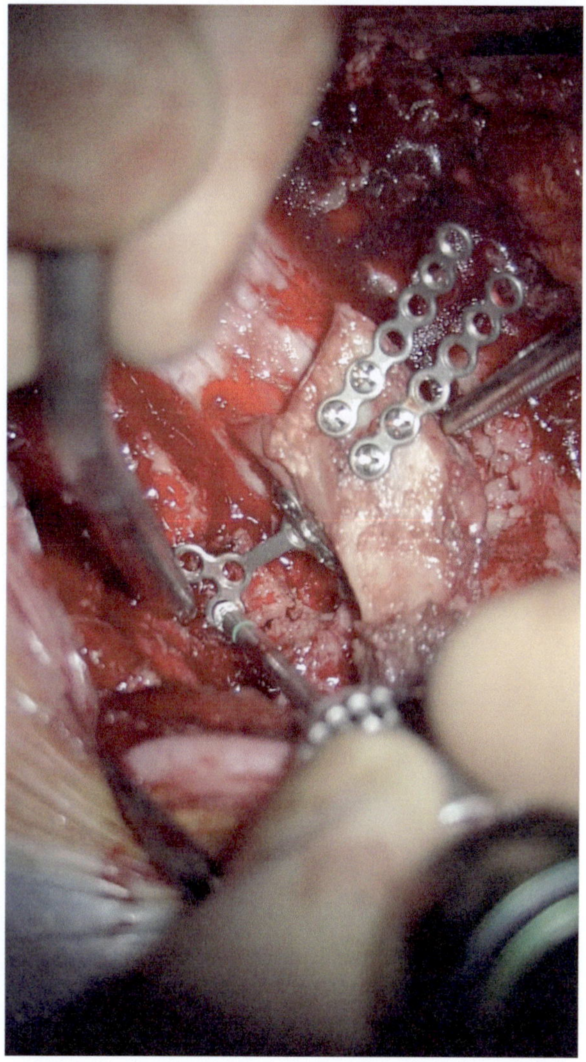

Fig. 8.52 Fixing of the lamina of C6 on the short side with small titanium plates

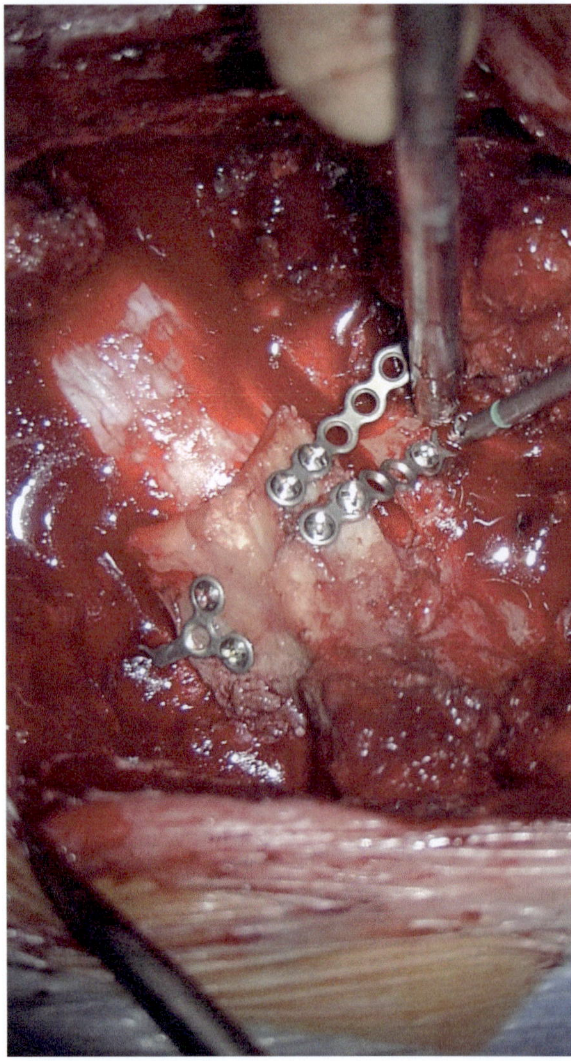

Fig. 8.53 Fixing of the lamina of C6 on the open side with longer titanium plates

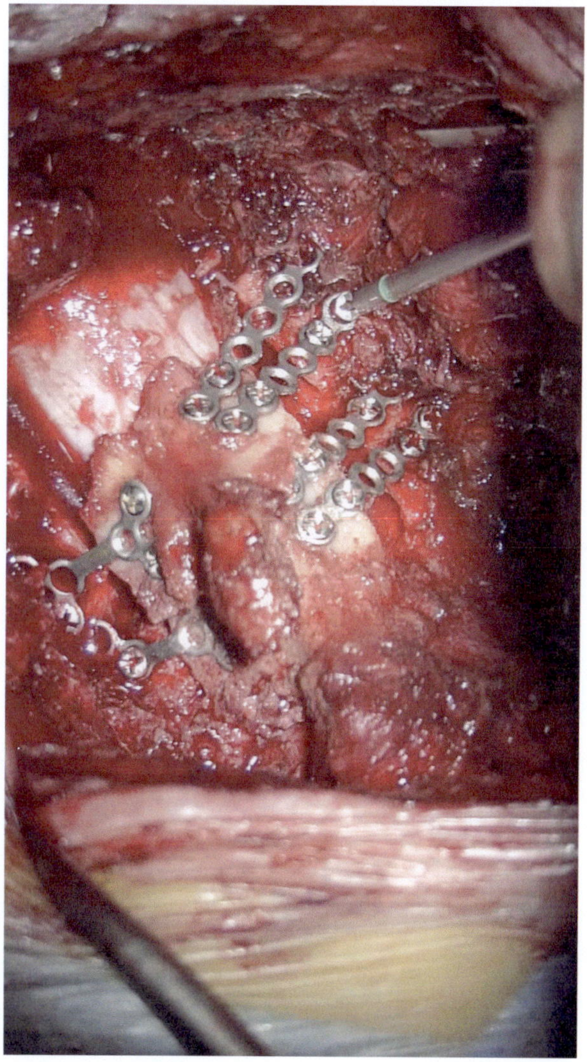

Fig. 8.54 Fixing of the lamina of C5 on the open side

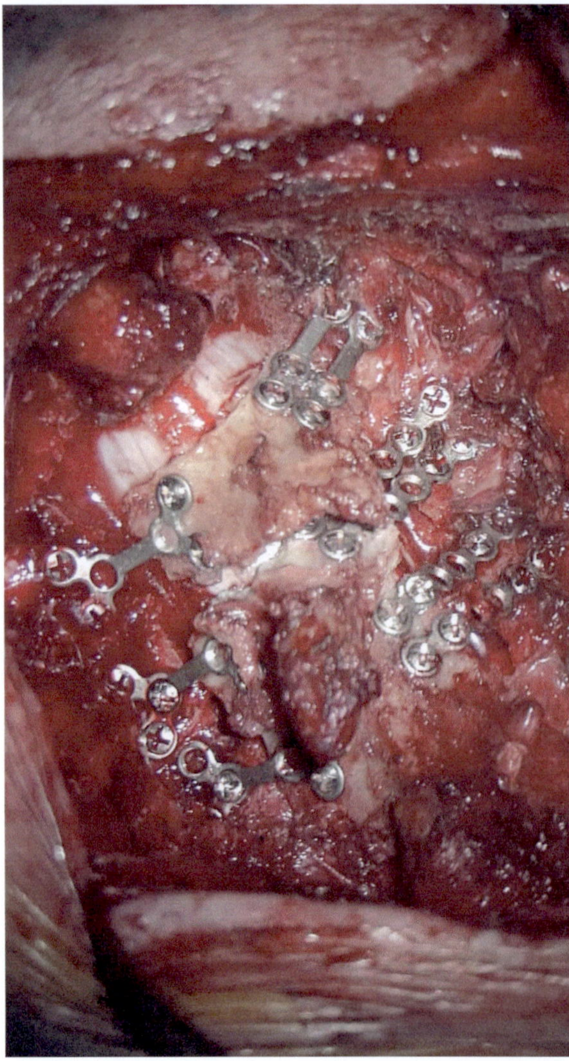

Fig. 8.55 Completed laminoplasty from C4 to C6

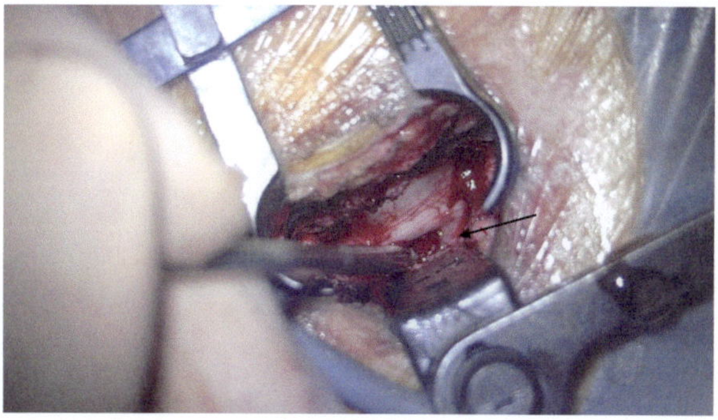

Fig. 8.56 Foraminotomy as described by Frykholm at the level C7/T1 on the left side. Minimal-invasive approach with a Piccolino™ retractor (Medicon, Tuttlingen, Germany). Situation after left-sided laminotomy of C7 and T1 with widening of the neuroforamen by using the undercutting technique for decompression of the C8 nerve root (*arrow*)

References

Caspar W, Barbier DD, Klara PM. Anterior cervical fusion and Caspar plate stabilization for cervical trauma. Neurosurgery. 1989;25(4):491–502.

Kim PK, Alexander JT. Indications for circumferential surgery for cervical spondylotic myelopathy. Spine J. 2006;6(6 Suppl):299S–307S.

Komotar RJ, Mocco J, Kaiser MG. Surgical management of cervical myelopa- thy: indications and techniques for laminectomy and fusion. Spine J. 2006;6(6 Suppl):252S–67S.

König SA, Ranguis S, Spetzger U. Management of complex cervical instability. J Neurol Surg A Cent Eur Neurosurg. 2013;76(2):119–25. doi:10.1055/s- 0033-1345095.

König SA, Spetzger U. Surgical management of cervical spondylotic myelopathy – indications for anterior, posterior or combined procedures for decompression and stabilisation. Acta Neurochir. 2014a;156(2):253–8.

König SA, Spetzger U. Modified open-door laminoplasty for the surgical treatment of cervical spondylotic myelopathy in elderly patients. Acta Neurochir. 2014b;156:1225–30.

Medow JE, Trost G, Sandin J. Surgical management of cervical myelopathy: indications and techniques for surgical corpectomy. Spine J. 2006;6(6 Suppl):233S–41S.

9 Information and Consent of the Patient

Due to the experiences with cervical spinal surgery for decades, the statistical risks of severe complications caused by an operation have significantly decreased. Nevertheless, the patient has to be informed about these risks, and this information has to be documented in a consent form. In general, the risks for severe complications (injury of the spinal cord or nerve roots or blood vessels as well as the trachea and oesophagus) lie in the field of single-digit percentage or even less than 1 %. The prognosis of remission of a radicular syndrome after surgical decompression is very good. Likewise the results after surgical decompression in cases of spondylotic myelopathy have significantly improved.

9.1 Outcome and Risks of Surgery

The main percentage of patients with cervical disc herniation shows cervicobrachialgia as the leading symptom, often accompanied by sensory disorders of the upper limb. The prognosis in terms of remission of these symptoms after surgery is very good. In cases of motor deficits, the prognosis is best in cases of short history and/or slight pareses.

The daily clinical practice shows that by an operation and the consecutive local decompression, a fast remission of pain is achieved that usually is sustained in the long term. Nevertheless, the patient has to be informed that due to progression of degeneration of one or more cervical levels, it is possible that symptoms reoccur.

For cervical spondylotic myelopathy, the preoperative prevalence of motor deficits of upper and lower limbs as well as sensory deficits of upper and lower limbs is higher than that of other disorders, whereas motor deficits of the lower limbs and sensory deficits of the lower limbs often persist after surgery (Machino et al. 2012). The risk of persisting damage of the spinal cord increases with higher age, smoking and/or vascular risk factors.

A. König, U. Spetzger, *Degenerative Diseases of the Cervical Spine*,
DOI 10.1007/978-3-319-47298-0_9

For the informed consent about surgery, there are special printed forms that were elaborated together by physicians and patients. These forms explain the surgical strategies and inform about the potential risks of surgery. Both should be discussed with and explained to the patient.

The worst complications during cervical spine surgery are of course injuries of the spinal cord, the main blood vessels, the trachea and the oesophagus as well as dislocations or breakout of implants (Bilbao et al. 2010; Saunders et al. 1998; Vaccaro et al. 1998). Further severe complications are CSF leaks, deep infections, secondary instability at the operated level and a palsy of the laryngeal recurrent nerve with hoarseness and dysphagia.

Implant-related complications can be heterotope ossification and pseudarthrosis at the operated level as well as accelerated adjacent level degeneration after fusion surgeries (Eleraky et al. 1999; Swank et al. 1997). General surgical risks include thrombosis, superficial wound healing disorder and keloid formation. The anaesthesiologist has to inform the patient about risks of anaesthesia.

If the harvesting of an iliac crest bone graft is indicated, the patient has to be informed about potential morbidity at the site of harvesting: haematoma, fracture and nerve injury.

Fehlings et al. (2012) analysed 302 cases that underwent either an anterior, posterior or circumferential procedure for the surgical treatment of cervical spondylotic myelopathy and detected a total complication rate of 15.6 %. The most frequent complications were cardiopulmonary events (3.0 %), dysphagia (3.0 %) and superficial wound healing disorder (2.3 %). A perioperative worsening of myelopathy was observed in 1.3 % of cases. In a follow-up after 2 years, the delayed complication rate was 4.4 %. Multivariate factors that were associated with a higher risk of complications were higher age, long operation time and combined approaches.

The incidence of intraoperative injury of the vertebral artery was quantified by Lunardi et al. (2013) with 0.07 % for all kinds of cervical spine surgeries. In 90 % the injury of the vertebral artery does not have permanent consequences for the patient. In 5.5 % it leads to persisting neurological deficits. Mortality was 4.5 %.

Zhu et al. (2013) found a significantly higher reoperation rate for anterior procedures (8.57 %) compared to posterior procedures (0.3 %) in a meta-analysis that included eight studies. Nevertheless, this meta-analysis showed a better recovery of myelopathy after anterior surgery than after posterior surgery.

For posterior fusions with lateral mass screws, Heller et al. (1995) found the following complication rates: injury of a nerve root in 0.6 %, injury of the spinal cord in 2.6 % and loosening of screws in 1.3 %.

In case of a radicular injury, the most frequent deficits are found for the C5 nerve root (Chiba et al. 2002; Tsuzuki et al. 1993). In patients with postoperative C5 palsy in half of the cases, a sensory deficit or pain in the C5 dermatome was observed. In the other half of cases, there was a weakness of the biceps muscle besides the weakness of the deltoid muscle (Yonenobu et al. 1991). The general incidence of postoperative C5 paresis is 4.6 % (Sakaura et al. 2003), whereas there are no significant differences between anterior (4.3 %) and posterior approach (4.7 %). A C5 injury is a serious complication for the patient since the deltoid muscle is innervated by this nerve root only. Thus, a C5 injury leads to a total loss of arm abduction which is a severe handicap in everyday life. Other muscles show only a partial weakness after monoradicular injury due to innervation by two or three nerve roots (e. g. the C5 and C6 innervation of the biceps brachii muscle).

For the therapy of the ossification of the posterior longitudinal ligament (OPLL), Smith et al. (2011) give detailed information about clinical outcome and complication rates in their study. A general neurological recovery 1 year after surgery was seen in 44 % in such a patient population according to a study by Kato et al. (1998). After anterior corpectomy for the treatment of OPLL in 15 % of cases, surgical revision is necessary due to pseudarthrosis (Epstein 1993, 1998). In cases of asymptomatic partial dislocation of cervical vertebral body replacement, it is possible to decide for a wait and see strategy with radiological follow-up examinations because most of those OPLL patients finally show a stable secondary fusion (Belanger et al. 2005; Choi et al. 2005).

References

Belanger TA, Roh JS, Hanks SE, et al. Ossification of the posterior longitudinal ligament. Results of anterior cervical decompression and arthrodesis in sixty-one North American patients. J Bone Joint Surg Am. 2005;87:610–5.

Bilbao G, Duart M, Aurrecoechea JJ, et al. Surgical results and complications in a series of 71 consecutive cervical spondylotic corpectomies. Acta Neurochir (Wien). 2010;152:1155–63.

Chiba K, Toyama Y, Matsumoto M, et al. Segmental motor paralysis after expansive open-door laminoplasty. Spine. 2002;27:2108–15.

Choi S, Lee SH, Lee JY, et al. Factors affecting prognosis of patients who underwent corpectomy and fusion for treatment of cervical ossification of the posterior longitudinal ligament: analysis of 47 patients. J Spinal Disord Tech. 2005;18:309–14.

Eleraky MA, Llanos C, Sonntag VK. Cervical corpectomy: report of 185 cases and review of the literature. J Neurosurg. 1999;90(1 Suppl):35–41.

Epstein N. The surgical management of ossification of the posterior longitudinal ligament in 51 patients. J Spinal Disord. 1993;6:432–55.

Epstein NE. Circumferential surgery for the management of cervical ossification of the posterior longitudinal ligament. J Spinal Disord. 1998;11:200–7.

Fehlings MG, Smith JS, Kopjar B, et al. Perioperative and delayed complications associated with the surgical treatment of cervical spondylotic myelopathy based on 302 patients from the AOSpine North America Cervical Spondylotic Myelopathy Study. J Neurosurg Spine. 2012;16(5):425–32.

Heller JG, Silcox III DH, Sutterlin III CE. Complications of posterior cervical plating. Spine. 1995;20:2442–8.

Kato Y, Iwasaki M, Fuji T, et al. Long-term follow-up results of laminectomy for cervical myelopathy caused by ossification of the posterior longitudinal ligament. J Neurosurg. 1998;89:217–23.

Lunardi DJ, Eskander MS, Even JL, et al. Vertebral artery injuries in cervical spine surgery. Spine J. 2013;S1529-9430(13):01556–8.

Machino M, Yukawa Y, Hida T, et al. The prevalence of pre- and postoperative symptoms in patients with cervical spondylotic myelopathy treated by cervical laminoplasty. Spine (Phila Pa 1976). 2012;37(22):E1383–8.

Sakaura H, Hosono N, Mukai Y, et al. C5 palsy after decompression surgery for cervical myelopathy: review of the literature. Spine. 2003;28:2447–51.

Saunders RL, Pikus HJ, Ball P. Four-level cervical corpectomy. Spine. 1998;23:2455–61.
Smith ZA, Buchanan CC, Raphael D, Khoo LT. Ossification of the posterior longitudinal ligament. pathogenesis, management, and current surgical approaches: a review. Neurosurg Focus. 2011;30(3):E10.
Swank ML, Lowery GL, Bhat AL, McDonough RF. Anterior cervical allograft arthrodesis and instrumentation: multilevel interbody grafting or strut graft reconstruction. Eur Spine J. 1997;6:138–43.
Tsuzuki N, Abe R, Saiki K, Okai K. Paralysis of the arm after posterior decompression of the cervical spinal cord. II. Analyses of clinical findings. Eur Spine J. 1993;2:197–202.
Vaccaro AR, Falatyn SP, Scuderi GJ, et al. Early failure of long segment anterior cervical plate fixation. J Spinal Disord. 1998;11:410–5.
Yonenobu K, Hosono N, Iwasaki M, et al. Neurologic complications of surgery for cervical compression myelopathy. Spine. 1991;16:1277–82.
Zhu B, Xu Y, Liu X, Liu Z, Dang G. Anterior approach versus posterior approach for the treatment of multilevel cervical spondylotic myelopathy: a systemic review and meta-analysis. Eur Spine J. 2013;22(7):1583–9.

Implant Safety and Complication Management

10

In cases of secondary dislocation of disc or vertebral body replacements, it is usually necessary to perform an anterior and/or posterior fusion during revision surgery. Material failure of cervical implants is observed very rarely. Especially in cases of osteoporosis, secondary subsidence of disc or vertebral body replacements is not an unusual complication. The aimed maintenance of motion after the relatively expensive total disc replacement can be completely neutralised by heterotopic ossification. The latter is evoked by excessive drilling during primary surgery. The implant safety of cages and prostheses has been significantly improved by stop devices at the insertion instruments. Complications like accidental injuries of the dura, blood vessels, trachea or oesophagus are usually treated surgically.

10.1 Dislocation of Implants

Dislocation of implants is observed after total disc replacement as well as vertebral body replacement (Figs. 10.1 and 10.2). Since there is always a damage to the adjacent endplates due to the removal of a dislocated prosthesis, it is not reasonable to reimplant a prosthesis because of the high risk of heterotopic ossification. The safest solution is a classical fusion with interposition of an iliac crest bone graft and additional anterior plating (Fig. 10.1).

10.2 Breaking of Implants

Nowadays, the cages, prostheses, plates and screws show a high measure of reliability due to ongoing biomechanical testing. In the lumbar spine, breaking of screws in overweight individuals is occasionally observed, but in the cervical spine, this is unlikely due to much less biomechanical stresses. It is more likely that screws

A. König, U. Spetzger, *Degenerative Diseases of the Cervical Spine*,
DOI 10.1007/978-3-319-47298-0_10

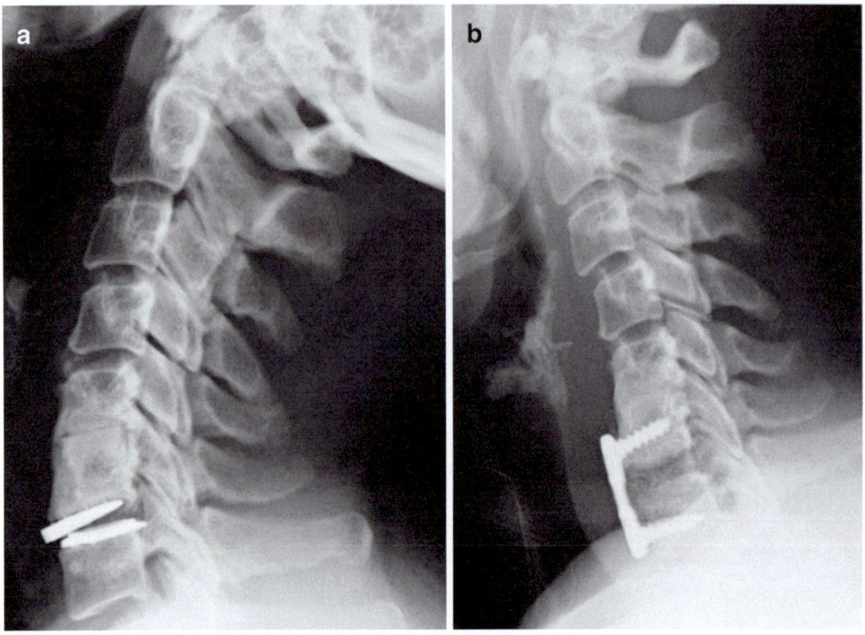

Fig. 10.1 Secondary dislocation of a cervical prosthesis Discover™, lateral X-ray image before (**a**) and after (**b**) revision surgery with interposition of an iliac crest bone graft and anterior plating. Both endplates of the partially dislocated implant showed bony fixation in the adjacent vertebral bodies and had to be removed by drilling out of the surrounding vertebral body

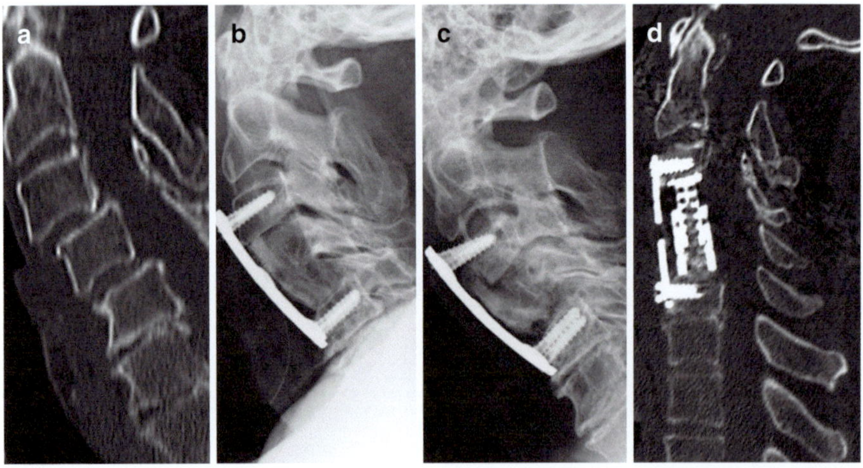

Fig. 10.2 Secondary surgical complication with breaking out of screws and dislocation of an iliac crest bone graft after anterior plating. Preoperative situation with degenerative instability, sagittal CT scan (**a**). Lateral X-ray image 1 day after surgery with adequate position of implants (**b**). Lateral X-ray image 3 months after surgery with breaking out of screws and dislocation of the bone graft (**c**). Sagittal CT scan after revision surgery with adjustable titanium vertebral body replacement ADD™ (**d**)

break out of the bone due to poor bone quality (Fig. 11.1c). In the authors' patient population of a few hundred individuals with cervical implants, there was only one case with a broken DCI implant after a car accident (Fig. 10.3). In such a case in the authors' opinion, it is reasonable to fuse the affected level analogue to cases of implant dislocation (Fig. 10.1) by using iliac crest bone graft and anterior plating.

10.3 Subsidence of Implants and Heterotopic Ossification

For total disc replacement, intact bony endplates of the adjacent vertebral bodies are a 'conditio sine qua non' for avoiding heterotopic ossification which would lead to a loss of function due to bony fusion of the relatively expensive implant. Therefore, the use of a drill has to be avoided when aiming total disc replacement. Nevertheless, heterotopic ossification occasionally occurs despite correct surgical technique (Fig. 10.4).

About the incidence of those undesirable events, there are different reports in the literature also depending on the type of prosthesis. Most clinical studies are still in progress (Richards et al. 2012).

For vertebral body replacement, the use of an autologous iliac crest bone graft is still the gold standard. If harvesting of an autologous bone graft is not possible for medical reasons, the implantation of a distractable titanium cage has proven to be of value. The use of a PEEK cage (Fig. 10.5) did not win recognition because of an increased of subsidence into adjacent vertebral bodies (König and Spetzger 2013).

In case of a subsided vertebral body replacement, it is often necessary to add a posterior fusion during revision surgery (Kim and Alexander 2006).

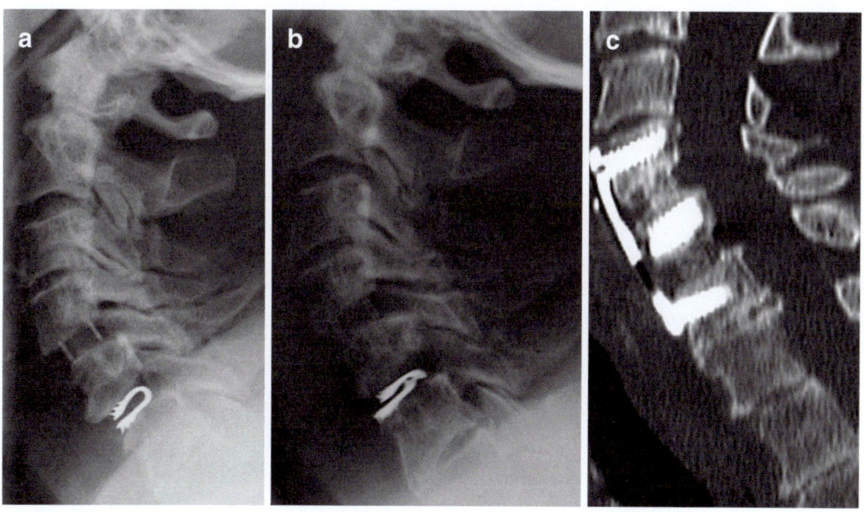

Fig. 10.3 Secondary breaking of a DCI implant after an accident. Primary surgery with cage fusion at C4/5 and DCI implant at C5/6, lateral X-ray image (**a**). Breaking of the DCI after a car accident with persisting neck pain, lateral X-ray image (**b**). Sagittal CT scan after revision surgery with replacement of the DCI by a PEEK cage and anterior plating (**c**)

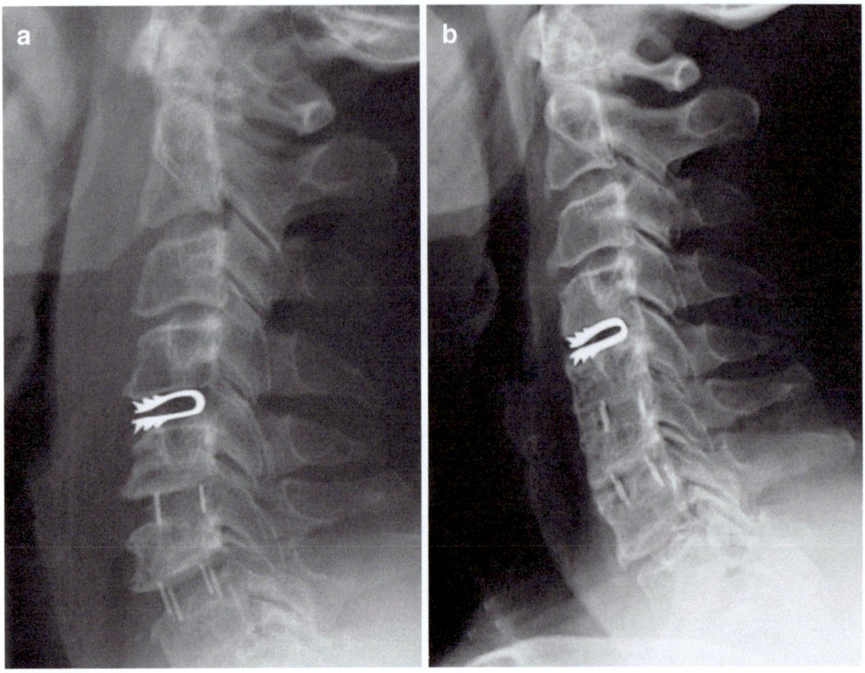

Fig. 10.4 Early postoperative lateral X-ray study after discectomy, decompression of the spinal canal and implantation of a DCI dynamic cervical implant at C4/5 and PEEK cages at C5/6 and C6/7 for the surgical treatment of spondylotic radiculopathy at these levels (**a**). Laterally X-ray study 2 years after surgery showing subsidence and posterior bony fusion of the DCI implant as well as intended bony fusion at C5/6 and C6/7 (**b**)

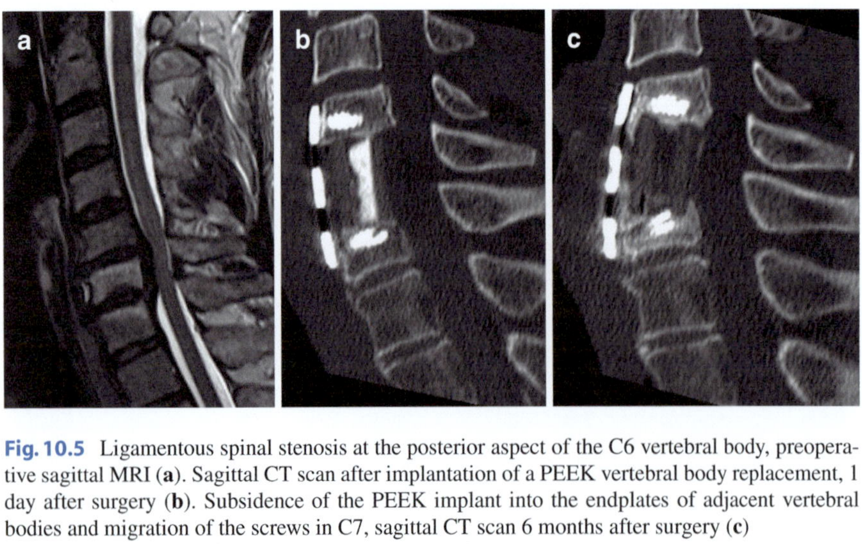

Fig. 10.5 Ligamentous spinal stenosis at the posterior aspect of the C6 vertebral body, preoperative sagittal MRI (**a**). Sagittal CT scan after implantation of a PEEK vertebral body replacement, 1 day after surgery (**b**). Subsidence of the PEEK implant into the endplates of adjacent vertebral bodies and migration of the screws in C7, sagittal CT scan 6 months after surgery (**c**)

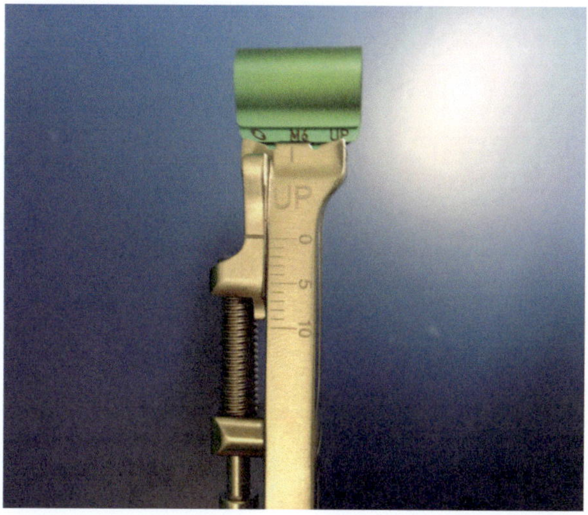

Fig. 10.6 Insertion tool for a DCI implant with adjustable stop device. Usually, the insertion depth is not adjusted beyond 3 mm

10.4 Implant Safety

The focus of discussion about implant safety has been on the insertion instruments for cages and prostheses since accidental posterior dislocation of an implant is possible during driving by impact with consecutive injury of the spinal cord. At the authors' institution, only cages and prostheses are used whose trial heads and insertion instruments have stop devices (Fig. 10.6) to avoid any complications during the implantation procedure. Safety for the patient is of first priority.

According to recent dispensation of justice in Germany, claims of compensation are possible in cases of complication due to missing stop devices at insertion instruments.

Furthermore, an implantation card documenting kind, localisation and serial number of the implant is mandatory (Figs. 10.7 and 10.8).

10.5 Product Liability

All of the used implant materials should be officially accredited products. They are subject to the Product Liability Act in Germany, and, thus, defectively produced and commercially distributed implants that cause damage to a patient's health are liable to pay damages. For personal injuries, the upper limit for compensation in the Product Liability Act currently is 85 million Euro. To which extent a material failure in a complex built prosthesis is a consequence of a problem during manufacturing or of a malpositioning during implantation will be difficult to prove in the individual case. For that specific problem, there is currently no dispensation of justice.

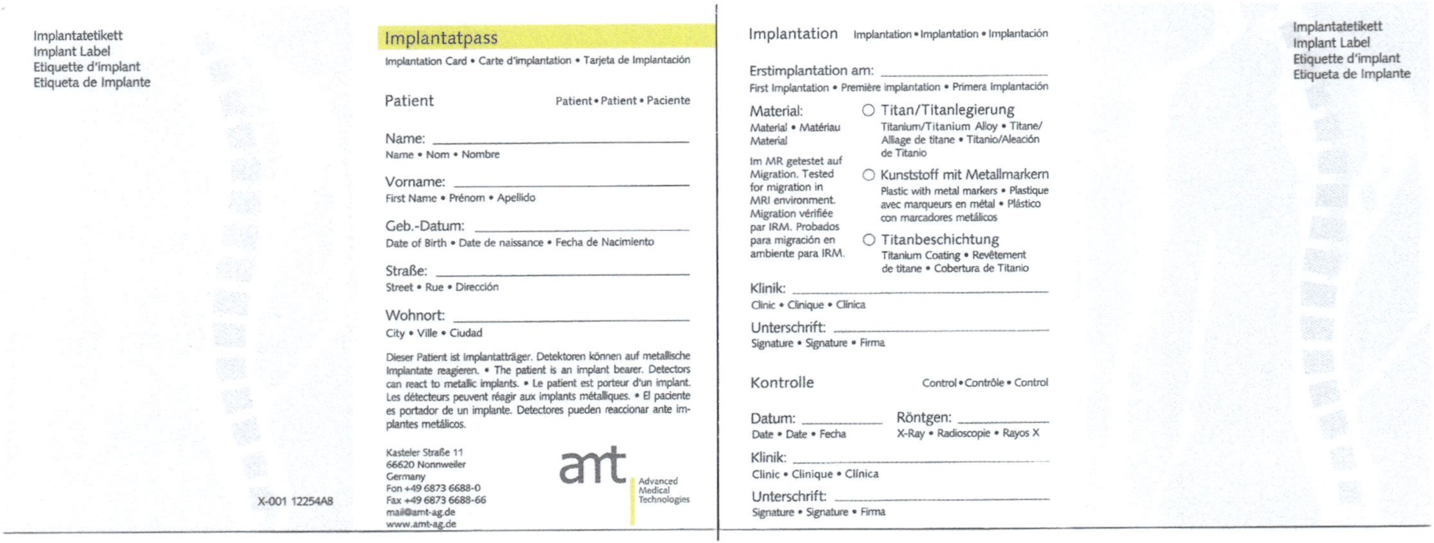

Implantatetikett
Implant Label
Etiquette d'implant
Etiqueta de Implante

X-001 12254AB

Implantatpass
Implantation Card • Carte d'implantation • Tarjeta de Implantación

Patient — Patient • Patient • Paciente

Name: ______
Name • Nom • Nombre

Vorname: ______
First Name • Prénom • Apellido

Geb.-Datum: ______
Date of Birth • Date de naissance • Fecha de Nacimiento

Straße: ______
Street • Rue • Dirección

Wohnort: ______
City • Ville • Ciudad

Dieser Patient ist Implantatträger. Detektoren können auf metallische Implantate reagieren. • The patient is an implant bearer. Detectors can react to metallic implants. • Le patient est porteur d'un implant. Les détecteurs peuvent réagir aux implants métalliques. • El paciente es portador de un implante. Detectores pueden reaccionar ante implantes metálicos.

Kasteler Straße 11
66620 Nonnweiler
Germany
Fon +49 6873 6688-0
Fax +49 6873 6688-66
mail@amt-ag.de
www.amt-ag.de

amt Advanced Medical Technologies

Implantation — Implantation • Implantation • Implantación

Erstimplantation am: ______
First Implantation • Première implantation • Primera Implantación

Material:
Material • Matériau
Material

Im MR getestet auf Migration. Tested for migration in MRI environment. Migration vérifiée par IRM. Probados para migración en ambiente para IRM.

○ Titan/Titanlegierung
Titanium/Titanium Alloy • Titane/Alliage de titane • Titanio/Aleación de Titanio

○ Kunststoff mit Metallmarkern
Plastic with metal markers • Plastique avec marqueurs en métal • Plástico con marcadores metálicos

○ Titanbeschichtung
Titanium Coating • Revêtement de titane • Cobertura de Titanio

Klinik: ______
Clinic • Clinique • Clínica

Unterschrift: ______
Signature • Signature • Firma

Kontrolle — Control • Contrôle • Control

Datum: ______
Date • Date • Fecha

Röntgen: ______
X-Ray • Radioscopie • Rayos X

Klinik: ______
Clinic • Clinique • Clínica

Unterschrift: ______
Signature • Signature • Firma

Implantatetikett
Implant Label
Etiquette d'implant
Etiqueta de Implante

Fig. 10.7 Example of an implantation card for a Shell™ cage by Advanced Medical Technologies

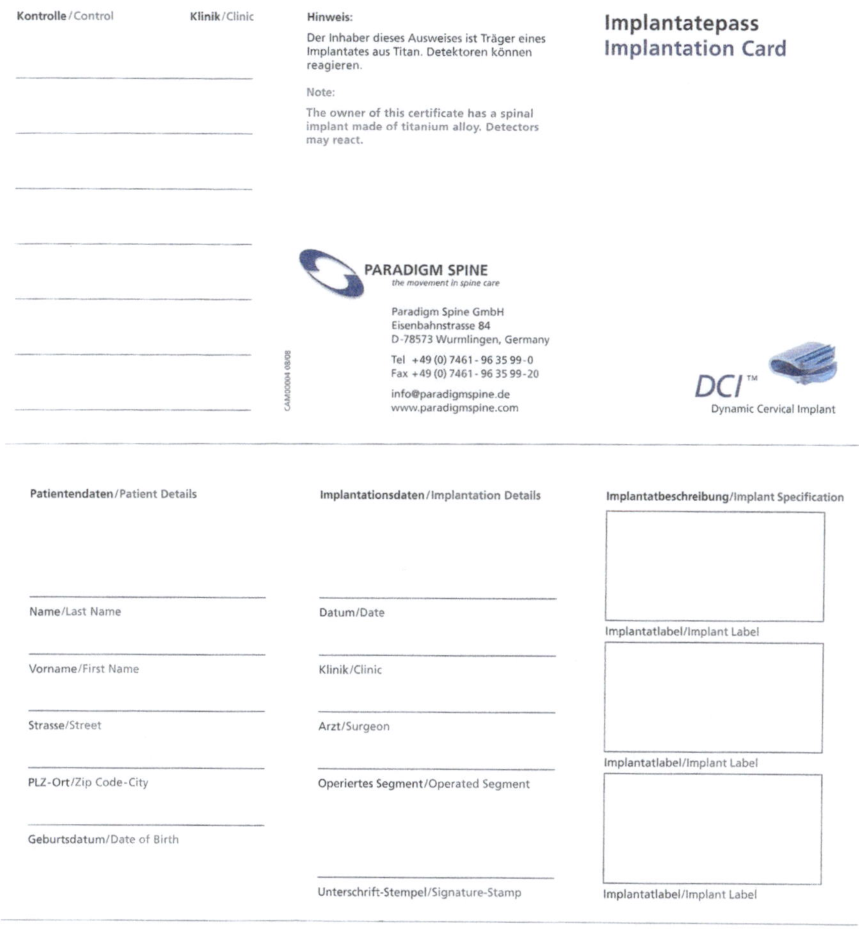
Kontrolle/Control Klinik/Clinic

Hinweis:
Der Inhaber dieses Ausweises ist Träger eines Implantates aus Titan. Detektoren können reagieren.

Note:
The owner of this certificate has a spinal implant made of titanium alloy. Detectors may react.

PARADIGM SPINE
the movement in spine care

Paradigm Spine GmbH
Eisenbahnstrasse 84
D-78573 Wurmlingen, Germany
Tel +49 (0) 7461 - 96 35 99 - 0
Fax +49 (0) 7461 - 96 35 99 - 20
info@paradigmspine.de
www.paradigmspine.com

Implantatepass
Implantation Card

DCI™
Dynamic Cervical Implant

Patientendaten/Patient Details
Name/Last Name
Vorname/First Name
Strasse/Street
PLZ-Ort/Zip Code-City
Geburtsdatum/Date of Birth

Implantationsdaten/Implantation Details
Datum/Date
Klinik/Clinic
Arzt/Surgeon
Operiertes Segment/Operated Segment
Unterschrift-Stempel/Signature-Stamp

Implantatbeschreibung/Implant Specification
Implantatlabel/Implant Label
Implantatlabel/Implant Label
Implantatlabel/Implant Label

Fig. 10.8 Example of an implantation card for a dynamic cervical implant (DCI) by Paradigm Spine

10.6 CSF Leak

In case of an intraoperative dural injury, it is recommended to immediately close the CSF leak by using USP 5–0 or 6–0 sutures under microscopic view. If it is not possible to achieve a watertight closure of the dura, it is recommended to use a fibrin glue or a Tachosil™ sealant patch (Takeda, Linz, Austria). The patch contains fibrinogen and thrombin, and when it is slightly pushed against the dura with a moistened surgical cotton ball, it permanently sticks to the dura. In cases of extensive defects or persisting CSF leak, it is recommended to add a lumbar CSF drainage. Persisting small dural injuries can be successfully treated by secondary application of a lumbar drainage. Persisting subcutaneous or percutaneous CSF leaks have to be surgically treated with the obligatory insertion of a lumbar drainage during revision surgery.

10.7 Vascular Complications

Venous bleedings while decompressing the neuroforamina after resection of the posterior longitudinal ligament occur relatively often. The first step is a tilting of the operating table with the upper part of the body being higher than the lower part of the body to reduce the intensity of the venous bleeding. Then the application of small absorbable gelatin sponges (Gelita-Spon by Gelita Medical, Eberbach, Germany) under irrigation often provides adequate haemostasis.

If these actions do not lead to haemostasis, the application of a haemostatic matrix (Floseal by Baxter, Unterschleißheim, Germany) is indicated. After application, the Floseal matrix has to be slightly pushed with surgical cotton balls.

A very rare complication during anterior cervical surgery is an injury of the common carotid artery that can be treated by an experienced surgeon by suturing. Alternatively, a vascular surgeon should be involved.

Injuries of the vertebral artery are difficult to treat in terms of preserving this blood vessel since it is mostly injured when removing bone in the uncinated recess with a drill or Kerrison punch. Due to the kind of injury to the vessel's wall in most cases, a packing is necessary. Sometimes the use of a clip as used in intracranial aneurysm surgery or a suture is successful. After surgery, an angiogram is indicated to rule out a pseudoaneurysm of the vertebral artery.

10.8 Injuries of the Trachea and Oesophagus

After accidental injury of the trachea or oesophagus, an ENT or visceral surgeon should be involved at an early stage to achieve sufficient suturing. After suturing the oesophagus, it is required to place a stomach tube for gavage for a few days. For documentation of a sufficient suture, a postoperative Barium swallow X-ray study is mandatory.

References

Kim PK, Alexander JT. Indications for circumferential surgery for cervical spondylotic myelopathy. Spine J. 2006;6(6 Suppl):299S–307S.

König SA, Spetzger U. Distractable titanium cages versus PEEK cages versus iliac crest bone grafts for the replacement of cervical vertebrae. Minim Invasive Ther Allied Technol. 2013;23(2):102–5.

Richards O, Choi D, Timothy J. Cervical arthroplasty: the beginning, the middle, the end? Br J Neurosurg. 2012;26(1):2–6.

The Future of Cervical Spine Surgery 11

On the basis of recent spine research, the manufacturing of individualised implants is possible. Using patient-specific computed tomography or magnetic resonance imaging data, an individual spine model can be rendered. With the help of such a model, an implant can be individually configured. Furthermore, it might be possible to test virtually the biomechanical behaviour of the cervical spine after implantation when using the finite element method. Another field of research is biological disc replacement by autologous transplantation of chondrocytes. At the thoracic and lumbar spines, the augmentation of screws with polymethylmethacrylate in cases of severe osteoporosis has been established for many years. Thus, this technique could be used for the cervical spine, too.

11.1 Benefit of Total Disc Replacement

Despite the numerous prostheses for total disc replacement available on the market, there is still ongoing discussion about and controversy over the benefit of these relatively expensive implants (Bae et al. 2015; Radcliff et al. 2015). In particular, the avoidance of adjacent degeneration is still the focus of research (Richards 2012). Furthermore, the follow-up intervals of most studies are relatively short, since most implants have been on the market for less than 10 years.

11.2 Autologous Chondrocyte Transplantation for Disc Replacement

In the future there will be probably a trend towards biological replacement using autologous chondrocytes. This might be an alternative to mechanical prostheses in total disc replacement. However, no valid data are available for this procedure. Case

A. König, U. Spetzger, *Degenerative Diseases of the Cervical Spine*,
DOI 10.1007/978-3-319-47298-0_11

reports and experiences have been gleaned from a phase I study of the lumbar spine. These results may lead to a useful and safe alternative to mechanical total disc replacement. However, valid results will likely not be available for years.

11.3 Augmentation of Screws in Fusion Cases

The use of augmented screws has been established in lumbar spine surgery for osteoporosis or revision cases. A pre-condition is the use of cannulated screws to enable the application of fluid polymethylmethacrylate (PMMA) into the cancellous bone. After the PMMA hardens, a tight junction between screws and the bone emerges.

Reports of PMMA augmentation in screwing the dens axis (Kohlhof et al. 2013) and in anterior plating of the cervical spine (Jo et al. 2012; Waschke et al. 2013) are available from small patient populations undergoing cervical surgery. We used PMMA augmentation for secondary breakout after anterior plating in patients with osteoporosis (Fig. 11.1). With increasing life expectancy, more and more patients with osteoporosis will likely have to be treated, and thus the number of cases with an indication for PMMA augmentation of screws will increase.

As mentioned in Chap. 7.2.2 page 67, the use of spreading screws did not win recognition since reports are available of increased breakout rates after using that kind of screw, even in patients without osteoporosis (König and Spetzger 2014).

The use of PMMA has also disadvantages, such as an exothermal hardening process and the release of toxic remnant monomers. Therefore the use of alternative substances and materials has been investigated (Hollstein 2003), but to date there are no noteworthy alternatives to PMMA.

11.4 Manufacturing and Implantation of an Individualised 3-Dimensional Printed Titanium Cage for Cervical Fusion

11.4.1 General Considerations

At present, anterior cervical discectomy and fusion (ACDF) with implantation of cages made of various biocompatible materials, with or without anterior plating, is the standard surgical treatment for spondylotic cervical myelopathy and/or radiculopathy (Cabraja et al. 2012; Kolstad et al. 2010; Wu et al. 2012; Yamagata et al. 2012).

The numerous cervical cages offered by the industry more or less mimic the anatomy of the intervertebral disc space, whereas the size and design of the cages are adapted to match the average shapes and sizes of a patient's intervertebral discs. The strategy of standalone cages without an additional plate reduces the invasiveness of the procedure and is gaining overall acceptance.

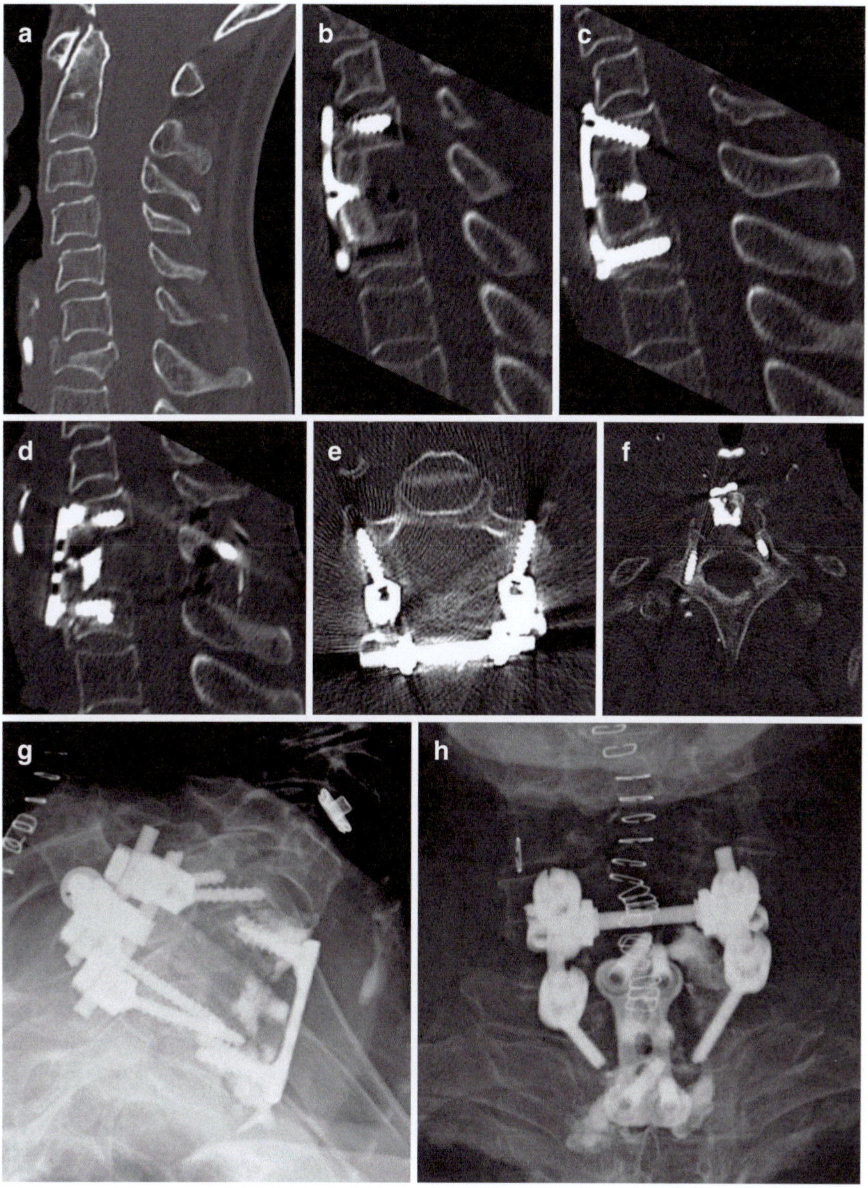

Fig. 11.1 Sagittal computed tomography (CT) scan showing a burst fracture of the C7 vertebra after a fall in an 80-year-old female patient (**a**). Postoperative sagittal CT scan 1 day after surgery showing the correct position of all implants (**b**). Sagittal CT scan showing the secondary breakout of screws in the C6 vertebral body (**c**). Situation after revision surgery with a shorter anterior plate and polymethylmethacrylate (PMMA) augmentation of the screws in C6 and T1 as well as posterior fusion of C6 to T1, as seen on sagittal (**d**) and axial (**e**, **f**) CT scans. Good visualisation of the PMMA material in lateral (**g**) and anteroposterior (**h**) radiography studies

The philosophy of our innovative project was to adapt a cage to a patient's individual anatomy and not – as usual – adapt the patient's anatomy to a commercially available cage. This development aims to create an implant that perfectly fits the individual endplates of the adjacent vertebral bodies in order to avoid fusion complications such as secondary dislocation or subsidence of the cage. Together with our industrial partners, we created a patient-specific and individualised cervical cage for ACDF.

This report summarises our interdisciplinary scientific industrial cooperation with computer-aided planning (virtual reality interactive simulation), manufacturing by 3-dimensional (3D) printing (selective laser melting) and surgical implantation of an individualised cervical cage. Simulation and planning were performed with 3D Systems, Rock Hill, SC. The manufacturing and 3D printing of the cage were performed by Emerging Implant Technologies GmbH (EIT), Tuttlingen, Germany. The surgical procedure was performed at the Department of Neurosurgery, Städtisches Klinikum Karlsruhe (SKK), Karlsruhe, Germany.

The first surgical procedure implanting such a customised 3D-printed cervical cage was performed in May 2015. A report of the whole project was published in 2016 in the *European Spine Journal* as a technical innovation (Spetzger et al. 2016).

11.4.2 Computer-Aided Planning and Virtual Reality Simulation

Using a DICOM CT data set (1.0-mm slice thickness), a 3D model of the patient's cervical spine is rendered ('rendered anatomy of the cervical spine'; Fig. 11.2). After analysing the 3D model with a focus on deformities, any kyphosis is virtually corrected by repositioning the C6 and C7 vertebrae ('repositioned anatomy'; Fig. 11.3). With this procedure the individualised cage obtains the ideal lordotic angle for restoring the sagittal balance of the cervical spine.

The next planning step is the virtual resection of osteophytes ('resected anatomy'; Fig. 11.4). The resection of posterior osteophytes is necessary to adequately decompress the spinal cord and nerve roots. The resection of anterior osteophytes should be considered if they obstruct the entrance to the disc space or especially in the case of symptomatic dysphagia.

Afterwards, the cage implantation can be simulated to check the implant's accuracy of fit ('implant placement'; Fig. 11.5). The height and facet joint orientation at adjacent levels must be considered when determining the optimum height of the implant. The planning starts with the existing data for an EIT standard titanium cage, which is modified according to the patient's individual anatomy. After rendering the individual shape of the of the patient's endplates, the final height of the implant is determined (Fig. 11.6). In the final stages, the entire virtual reality simulation and planning process is interactively modified and reviewed by the neurosurgeon. This last step finalises the definitive form of the cage before it goes into production.

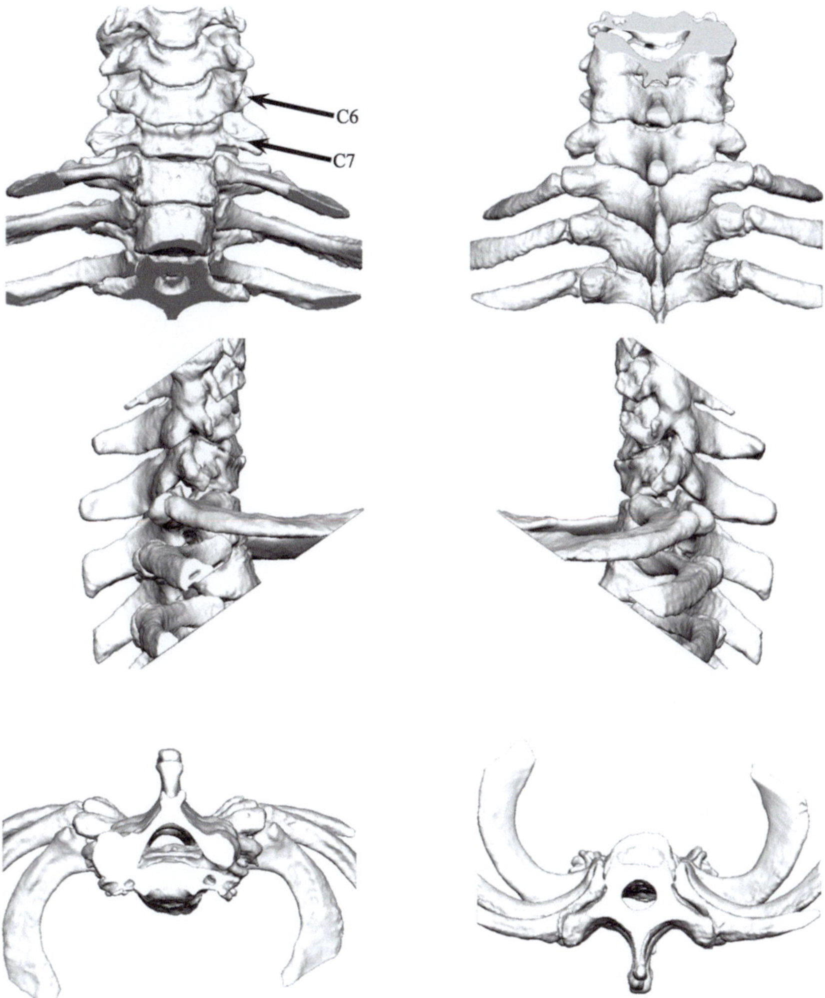

Fig. 11.2 3-Dimensional volume rendering of a patient's computed tomography data set showing the anatomic conditions with degeneration at C6–7 and slight kyphosis

11.4.3 Manufacturing

EIT manufactures the porous titanium cage slice by slice using selective laser melting, a modern additive production process. During this process, a very thin layer of titanium alloy powder, in this case TiAl6V4, is applied to a base plate. The titanium alloy powder is completely melted by a laser beam and forms a tight layer after consolidation. After this process, the base plate is lowered 30–50 µm, and the next layer is applied. This procedure is repeated until all layers are completed and the cage achieves its final shape. Additionally, it is possible to mimic

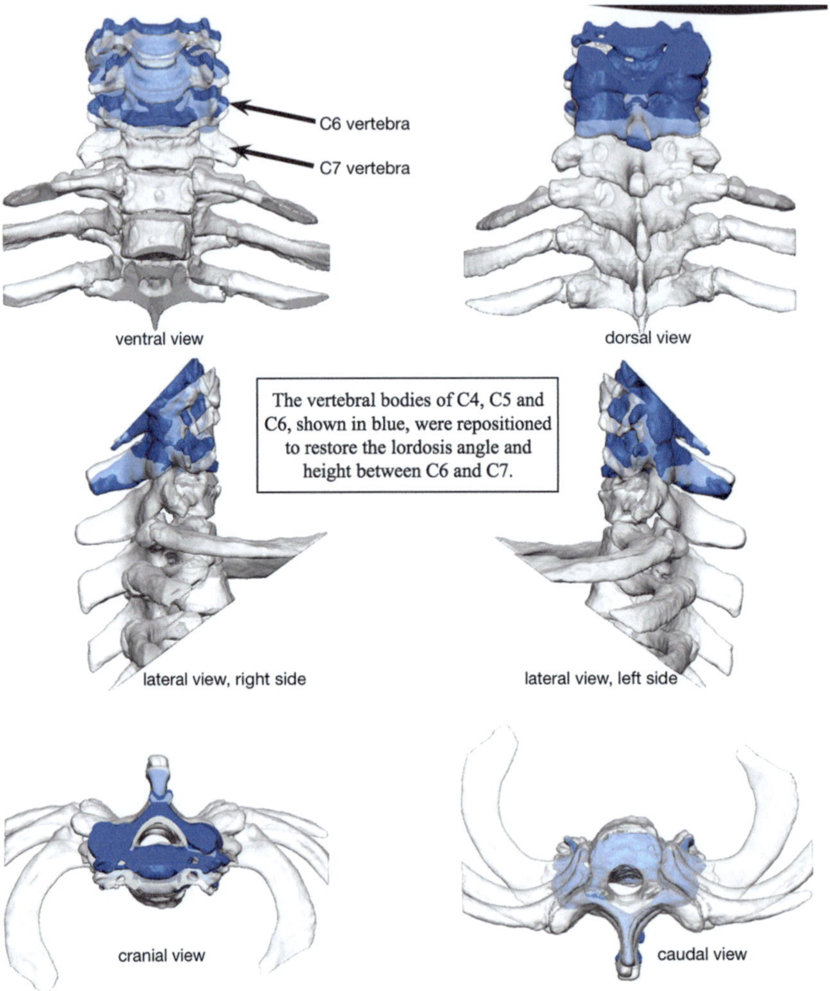

Fig. 11.3 Repositioned anatomy with virtual correction of the patient's spondylotic kyphosis

the trabecular structure of bone inside a titanium fusion cage. The cage is made of EIT Cellular Titanium with 80 % porosity and a pore size of 0.65 mm, which provides good pre-conditions for secondary bony fusion without an additional synthetic bone graft (Fig. 11.7).

The laser beam is guided by special 3D computer-assisted design software that divides the device into several layers and calculates the lanes of the laser. On the basis of the patient's particular 3D data set, the pre-calculated 3D form of the cage is precisely replicated and shows the exact anatomy of the patient's individual disc space (Fig. 11.7).

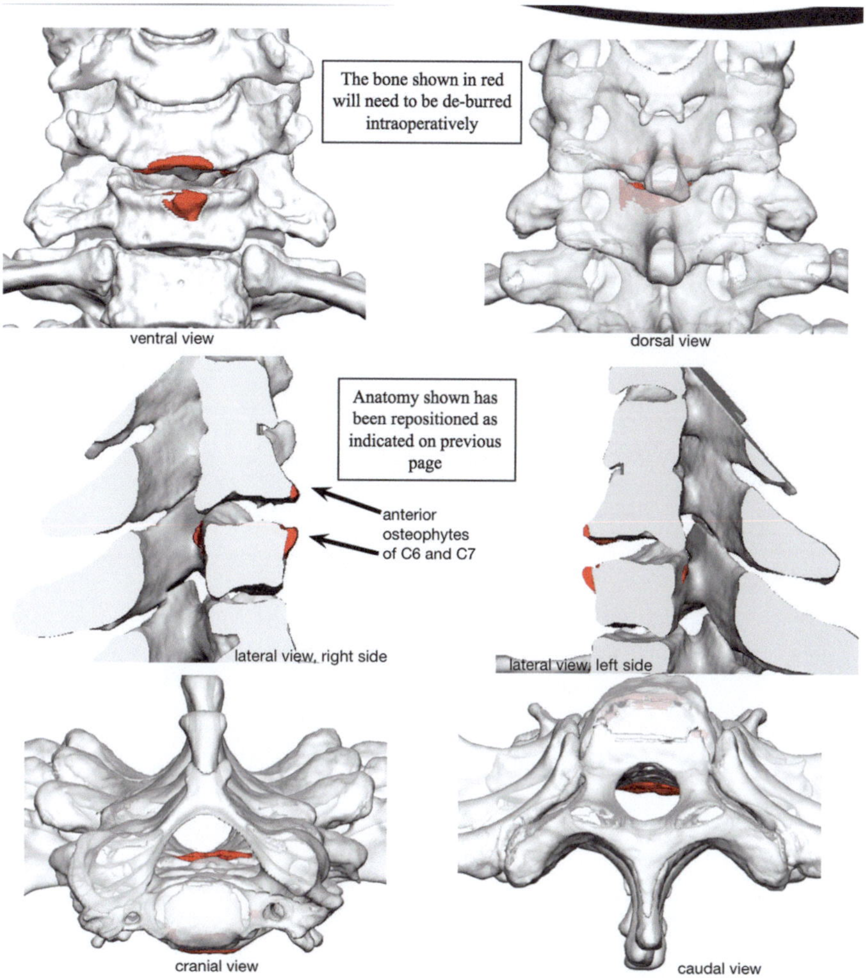

Fig. 11.4 'Virtual surgical procedure'. The simulation shows the osteophytes that need to be resected during surgery

11.4.4 Surgical Implantation

For ACDF with decompression, we use the standard anterolateral approach to the level C6–7 of the cervical spine. First, anterior osteophytes are resected as virtually planned, followed by discectomy and microsurgical decompression of the cervical spinal canal and the foramina. Posterior osteophytes that narrow the spinal canal and the foramina are selectively removed with a 4 mm the diameter of the drill or a 2 mm the diameter of the punch under a microscope. We avoid damaging the bony endplates of the adjacent vertebral bodies to allow a perfect fit for the cage and to prevent subsidence. The final step is implanting the cage using intraoperative

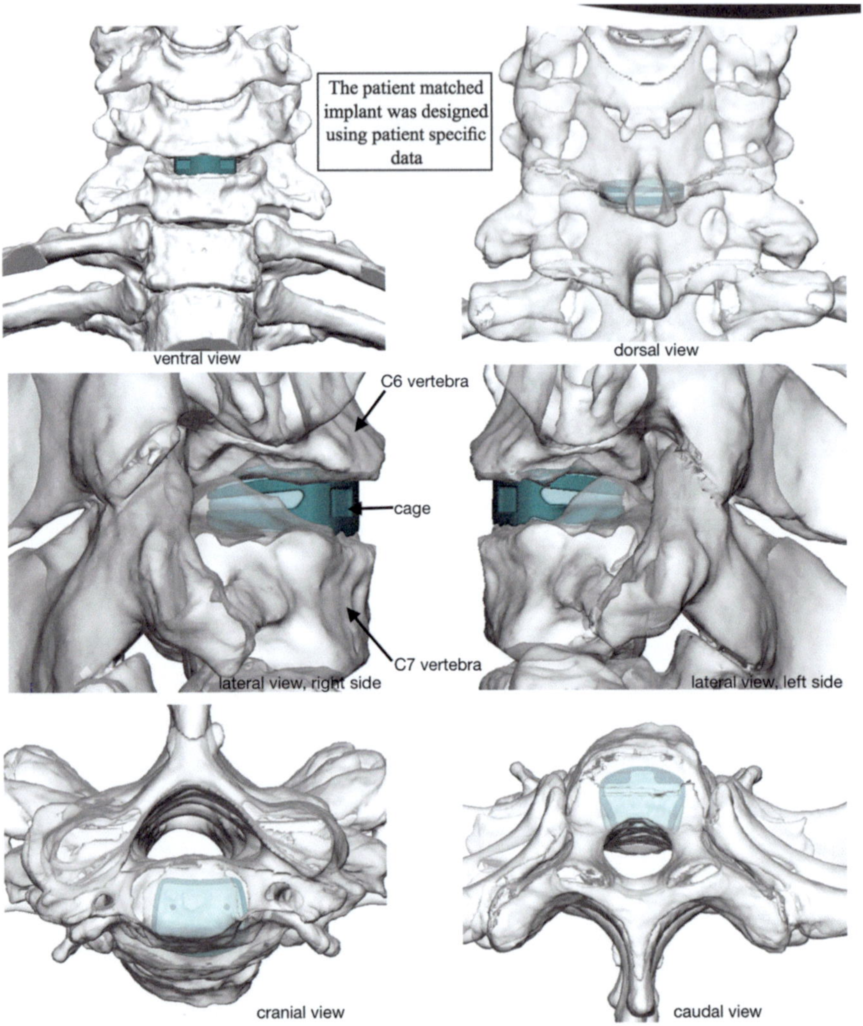

Fig. 11.5 Virtual reality planning and simulation of the implant position and design according to the patient's individual anatomy

fluoroscopy. A Caspar retractor is slightly over-distracted for the implantation of the 3D-printed cage. The cage thereby 'finds' its correct position after suspending distraction through its unique and perfectly fitting endplate design (Fig. 11.8). Furthermore, it is impossible to move the cage in any direction with the inserting instrument after suspending distraction, for the same reason.

The pilot project of the first-ever implantation of an individualised 3D-printed cervical cage resulted in a high accuracy of fit of the implant (Fig. 11.8). Thus, it can be assumed that an individualised cervical implant provides excellent

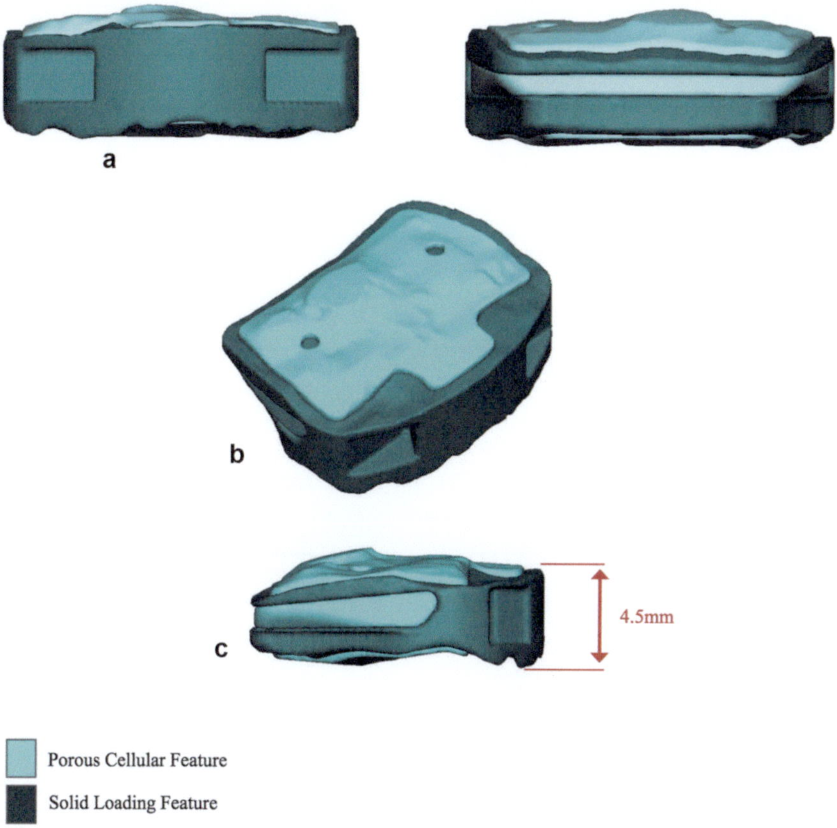

Fig. 11.6 Final design of the individual implant (anteroposterior view (**a**), oblique view (**b**)) demonstrates the individualised surface of the cage exactly mimicking the anatomy of the patient's endplates. (**c**) A lateral view shows the 4.5-mm measurement of the ventral disc height

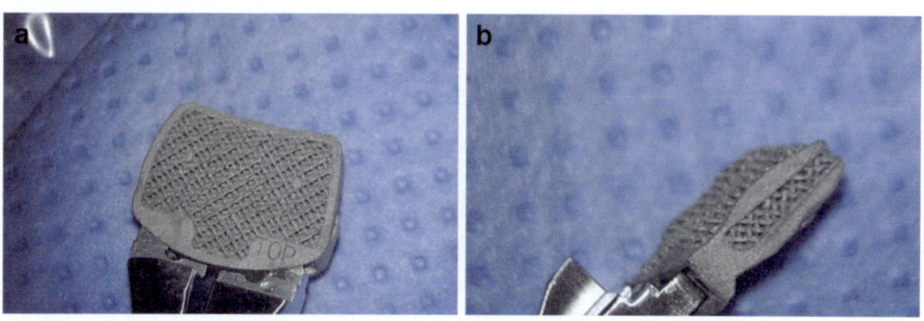

Fig. 11.7 The 3-dimensionally printed implant with a porous macro- and microcellular trabecular structure for improved osteointegration. (**a**) Top view of the individualised cage. (**b**) The lateral view demonstrates the irregular configuration of the patient's individual disc anatomy

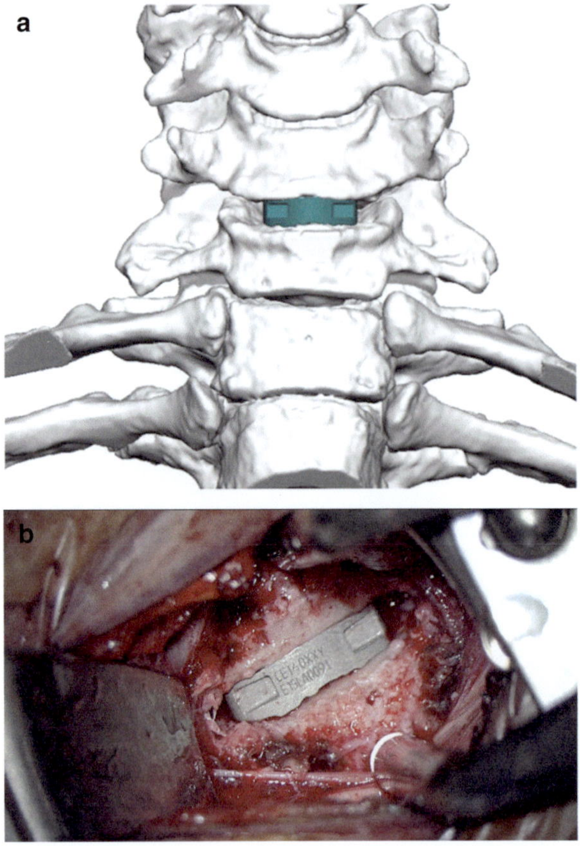

Fig. 11.8 (**a**) Virtual surgical planning and implantation of the 3-dimensional cage model. (**b**) Intraoperative photograph showing the perfect fit of the individualised titanium cage in situ after implantation, exactly corresponding to the virtual reality simulation and planning

primary stability. The final position of the cage is checked by intraoperative fluoroscopy after removing the distractor and pins. The perfect result is documented immediately postoperatively by anteroposterior and lateral radiography (Fig. 11.9).

11.4.5 Perspective

In summary, we present the technical preconditions for planning and manufacturing individualised 3D-printed cervical fusion cages using specific patient data. The implantation of these cages is as uncomplicated as the implantation of standard cages. Whether the improved load-bearing surface is able to reduce the rate of implant dislocation and cage subsidence should be evaluated in the future. Reasonably priced individualised 3D-printed cages must be developed by further collaboration between spine surgeons and industrial partners. However, the era of virtual reality in surgery, as well as 3D printing in surgery, has just begun (Spetzger et al. 2013).

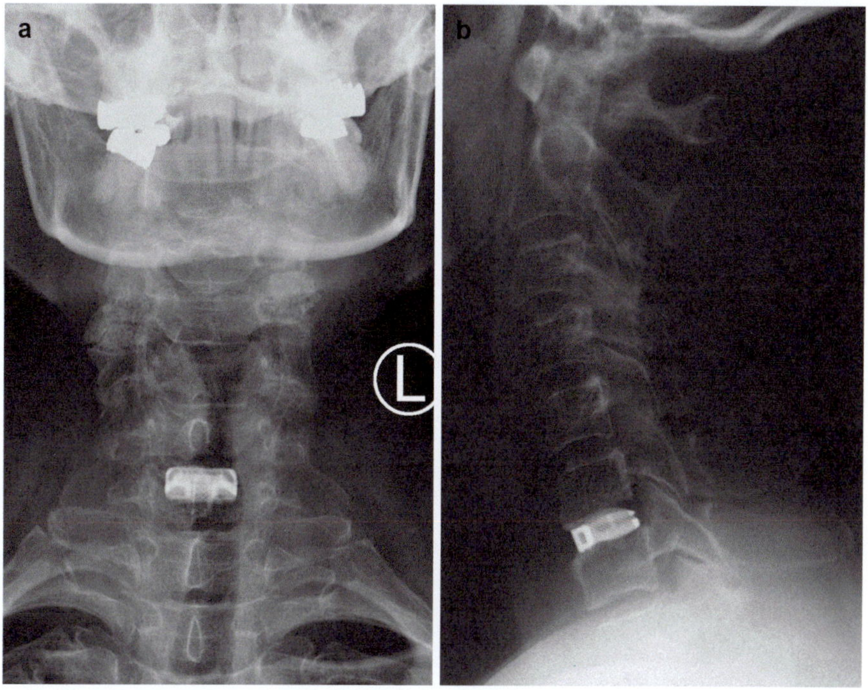

Fig. 11.9 Postoperative radiographic images after anterior cervical discectomy and fusion showing the fit of the implanted individualised 3-dimensionally printed titanium cage. The anteroposterior (**a**) and lateral (**b**) views confirm the perfect restored height and re-angulation of the disc space, exactly as preoperatively planned and simulated in virtual reality (compare with Fig. 11.4)

References

Bae HW, Kim KD, Nunley PD, Jackson RJ, Hisey MS, Davis RJ, Hoffman GA, Gaede SE, Danielson 3rd GO, Peterson DL, Stokes JM, Araghi A. Comparison of clinical outcomes of one and two-level total disc replacement: 4-year results from a prospective, randomized, controlled. Multicenter IDE Clinl Trial Spine (Phila Pa 1976). 2015;40(11):759–66.

Cabraja M, Oezdemir S, Koeppen D, Kroppenstedt S. Anterior cervical discectomy and fusion: comparison of titanium and polyetheretherketone cages. BMC Musculoskelet Disord. 2012;13:172.

Hollstein EP. Knöcherne Integration und Biokompatibilität eines neuen resorbierbaren Polymers zur Schraubenaugmentation im osteoporotischen Knochen. Dissertation, LMU München: Tierärztliche Fakultät; 2003.

Jo JY, Kang SH, Park SW. Modified polymethylmethacrylate cervical plate and screw augmentation technique for intraoperative screw loosening. J Spinal Disord Tech. 2012;25(4):235–9.

Kohlhof H, Seidel U, Hoppe S, et al. Cement-augmented anterior screw fixation of type II odontoid fractures in elderly patients with osteoporosis. Spine J. 2013;13(12):1858–63.

Kolstad F, Nygaard ØP, Andresen H, Leivseth G. Anterior cervical arthrodesis using a "stand alone" cylindric titanium cage: prospective analysis of radiographic parameters. Spine (Phila Pa 1976). 2010;35(16):1545–50.

König SA, Spetzger U. Distractable titanium cages versus PEEK cages versus iliac crest bone grafts for the replacement of cervical vertebrae. Minim Invasive Ther Allied Technol. 2014;23(2):102–5.

Radcliff K, Zigler J, Zigler J. Costs of cervical disc replacement versus anterior cervical discectomy and fusion for treatment of single-level cervical disc disease: an analysis of the blue health intelligence database for acute and long-term costs and complications. Spine (Phila Pa 1976). 2015;40(8):521–9.

Richards O, Choi D, Timothy J. Cervical arthroplasty: the beginning, the middle, the end? Br J Neurosurg. 2012;26(1):2–6.

Spetzger U, Schilling AV, Winkler G, Wahrburg J, König A. The past, present and future of minimally invasive spine surgery: a review and speculative outlook. Minim Invasive Ther Allied Technol. 2013;22(4):227–41.

Spetzger U, Frasca M, König SA. Surgical planning, manufacturing and implantation of an individualized cervical fusion titanium cage using patient-specific data. Eur Spine J. 2016;25(7):2239–46.

Waschke A, Walter J, Duenisch P, et al. Anterior cervical intercorporal fusion in patients with osteoporotic or tumorous fractures using a cement augmented cervical plate system: first results of a prospective single-center study. J Spinal Disord Tech. 2013;26(3):E112–7.

Wu WJ, Jiang LS, Liang Y, Dai LY. Cage subsidence does not, but cervical lordosis improvement does affect the long-term results of anterior cervical fusion with stand-alone cage for degenerative cervical disc disease: a retrospective study. Eur Spine J. 2012;21(7):1374–82.

Yamagata T, Takami T, Uda T, Ikeda H, Nagata T, Sakamoto S, Tsuyuguchi N, Ohata K. Outcomes of contemporary use of rectangular titanium stand-alone cages in anterior cervical discectomy and fusion: cage subsidence and cervical alignment. J Clin Neurosci. 2012;19(12):1673–8.

Index

A. König, U. Spetzger, *Degenerative Diseases of the Cervical Spine*,
DOI 10.1007/978-3-319-47298-0

FSC
www.fsc.org
MIX
Papier aus verantwortungsvollen Quellen
Paper from responsible sources
FSC® C105338

If you have any concerns about our products,
you can contact us on
ProductSafety@springernature.com

In case Publisher is established outside the EU,
the EU authorized representative is:
Springer Nature Customer Service Center GmbH
Europaplatz 3, 69115 Heidelberg, Germany

Printed by Libri Plureos GmbH
in Hamburg, Germany